V. GULIELMOS (ED.)

**Beating Heart Bypass Surgery
and Minimally Invasive Conduit Harvesting**

V. GULIELMOS (ED.)

Beating Heart Bypass Surgery and Minimally Invasive Conduit Harvesting

▌ Cardiosurgical Techniques
▌ Anesthesia Management

With 38 Figures and 15 Tables

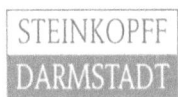

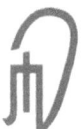

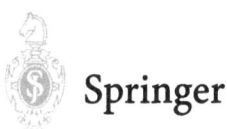

Prof. Dr. Vassilios Gulielmos
Geniki Kliniki Thessaloniki
Gravias 2, Paraliaki Ave.
54645 Thessaloniki
Greece

ISBN 978-3-7985-1399-0   ISBN 978-3-7985-1929-9 (eBook)
DOI 10.1007/978-3-7985-1929-9

Bibliographic information published by Die Deutsche Bibliothek
Die Deutsche Bibliothek lists this publication in the Deutsche Nationalbibliografie; detailed bibliographic data is available in the Internet at <http://dnb.ddb.de>.

http://www.steinkopff.springer.de

© Springer-Verlag Berlin Heidelberg 2004

Originally published by Steinkopff Verlag Darmstadt in 2004

Medical Editor: S. Ibkendanz   Production Manager: Thomas Tschech
Cover designer: Erich Kirchner, Heidelberg
Typesetter: K+V Fotosatz GmbH, Beerfelden

SPIN 10919576   85/7231-5 4 3 2 1 0 – Printed on acid-free paper

Preface

The 1970s and 1980s were the "golden years" of cardiac surgery, as the surgeons were the only ones to offer an alternative for the treatment of coronary artery disease. When catheter-based cardiovascular procedures appeared, not only did the overall number of cardiac interventions grow rapidly, but it also established itself as the minimally invasive alternative. As a consequence, the patient population for surgery started to change as well. It was not until the 1990s when surgery, with the introduction of less and minimally invasive techniques, stimulated also by other specialties (e.g. OB/GYN, urology), made a "come back". Various procedures in cardiac surgery were on the way of being performed minimally invasively. Whether it was valve replacements or repairs, septal defects, the coronaries or even tumors, all were refined. In this book, we focus on the minimally invasive coronary methods and all direct or indirectly related techniques.

Establishing new methods always takes time; it needs the pioneers and the early adopters to fine tune and bring them into our daily routine. Nonetheless, industry plays an equal role, with the pioneers on their side to bring the right devices for the new techniques. While the surgical products for OPCAB quickly became better and better, the adoption from the surgical side was lagging behind. Therefore, the question became how to convince our colleagues to use this new method. Exactly at this point and initiated by an industry representative, we started in Germany with "OPCAB Round Tables" where cardiac surgeons, anesthesiologists, cardiologists and perfusionists sat down with the industry to discuss the pro's and con's, the strengths and possible improvements, and the needs for OPCAB. After a few of those events the idea was born to place all of these ideas and "not yet" standards into a broader scope, into the book you are now holding in your hands.

The today more or less mature version of the "novel" techniques are described in order to help new users of minimal and less invasive cardiac surgery to avoid the mistakes and pitfalls already made and to help them start using it in the daily routine. The techniques are faster, more effective, simple and safe for the cardiac surgeon, but above all for our patients and their families.

This book would not have been possible without all of my colleagues and my scientific co-worker Ms Monika Weber standing behind it and supporting it along the way. A special thanks to Mr. Thomas Blauen who not only was instrumental in initiating but also in coordinating the logistics of this project along the way.

Thessaloniki (Greece), September 2003   VASSILIOS GULIELMOS

List of Contents

▌ Chapter 3: MIDCAB

▌ Chapter 4: Minimally Invasive Conduit Harvesting

List of Contributors

Dr. BERTHOLD BEIN
Department of Anaesthesiology
and Intensive Care Medicine
University Hospital Kiel
Schwanenweg 21
24105 Kiel
Germany

Dr. JOCHEN BÖRGERMANN
Department of Cardiac
and Thoracic Surgery
Martin-Luther-University
Halle-Wittenberg
Ernst-Grube-Str. 40
06120 Halle/Saale
Germany

Prof. Dr. JOCHEN CREMER
Department of
Cardiovascular Surgery
Christian Albrecht University
Arnold-Heller-Str. 7
24105 Kiel
Germany

Dr. RUUD COPPOOLSE
Department of Cardiac Surgery
Schüchtermann-Klinik
Ulmenallee 11
49214 Bad Rothenfelde
Germany

Dr. CHRISTIAN DETTER
Department of
Cardiovascular Surgery
University Hospital
Hamburg-Eppendorf
Martinistr. 52
20246 Hamburg
Germany

Dr. ANNO DIEGELER
Department of Cardiac Surgery
Cardiovascular Clinic
Salzburger Leite 1
97616 Bad Neustadt/Saale
Germany

Priv.-Doz. Dr. IVAR FRIEDRICH
Cardiothoracic Surgery
Martin Luther University Halle
06097 Halle
Germany

Prof. Dr. VASSILIOS GULIELMOS
Geniki Kliniki Thessaloniki
Gravias 2, Paraliaki Ave.
54645 Thessaloniki
Greece

Dr. JAN F. GUMMERT
Herzzentrum Leipzig
Struempellstr. 39
04289 Leipzig
Germany

Dr. KAVOUS HAKIM
Herzzentrum Coswig
Lerchenfeld 1
06869 Coswig
Germany

Dr. UTZ KAPPERT
Department of Cardiac Surgery
Heart Center Dresden
University Hospital
Fetscherstr. 76
01307 Dresden
Germany

Dr. ANTHOS KAPSALIS
Department of Cardiac Surgery
Heart Center Dresden
University Hospital
Fetschertr. 76
01307 Dresden
Germany

Dr. RONALD H. MILES
Wausau Heart & Lung Surgeons
425 Pine Ridge Blvd., Suite 209
Wausau, Wisconsin 54401
USA

Dr. JOACHIM NICOLAI
Department of
Cardiac Anesthesiology
Heart Center Dresden
University Hospital
Fetscherstr. 76
01307 Dresden
Germany

Dr. ARNO NIERICH
Isala Clinics
Department of Cardiothoracic
Anaesthesia & Intensive Care
Groot Wezenland 20
8000 GM Zwolle
The Netherlands

Dr. ULRICH ROSENDAHL
Department of Cardiothoracic
and Vascular Surgery
Heart Center Lahr/Baden
Hohbergweg
77933 Lahr
Germany

Dr. INA SCHADE
Department of Cardiac Surgery
Heart Center Dresden
University Hospital
Fetscherstr. 76
01307 Dresden
Germany

CHAPTER **1** **Introduction**

A historical review:
From standardized coronary bypass grafting to off-pump surgery

A. Diegeler

The development of modern cardiac surgery was initiated by the development of the heart-lung machine by Gibbon in 1954 [11]. Extracorporeal circulation ensured the supply of oxygenated blood to all organs except the heart and allowed surgery to be performed on the inside of the heart, i.e., on the valves and septums. The development of protective procedures for the heart itself, which is not supplied with blood during this kind of surgery, led to increased safety and further standardization of these surgical procedures. We have to point out at this point that the origins of cardiac surgery lie in the treatment of congenital malformations and heart valve defects, in particular in the area of rheumatic valve alterations. Only much later, during the further development of this young surgical discipline the search began for a method to treat widespread coronary heart diseases. Between 1955 and 1964, there were only sporadic reports of operations on the coronary arteries by Murray, Garrett, Sabiston and Longmire [10, 17, 21, 24]. Only after the cardiological working group of Effler and Sones [8] at the Cleveland Clinic was able to determine coronary artery disease (CAD) by the systematic development of coronary angiography was it possible to standardize surgical strategies. It was left to Favaloro [9] to introduce coronary bypass surgery as a therapy concept for the treatment of CAD in a standardized form. Within the scope of this kind of surgery, sternotomy as an access to the heart, the use of the heart-lung machine, moderate hypothermia for myocardial protection, and coronary revascularization by aorto-coronary vein bypasses became the standard. As late as 1970, this strategy was expanded by the use of the left internal mammary artery for revascularization of the left anterior descending artery (LAD) in the works of LOOP and coworkers [18]. With the further development of surgical techniques including extracorporeal perfusion, cardiac anesthesia and post-operative intensive care of the patients, the surgical revascularization concept of aorto-coronary bypass grafts for the revascularization of local coronary artery diseases was able to establish itself with high efficiency and safety. In the 1980s and 1990s, this surgical technique led to a boom, since systematic diagnostics using coronary angiography became a widespread tool. With the introduction of angioplasty by GRUENTZIG [12] in 1967, another pillar was formed for the treatment of coronary artery disease which has ever since competed with the surgical procedures. Especially due to the introduction of stents, several new methods for the treatment of in-stent stenoses which could not be removed previously and better drug treatments to avoid early occlusions, angioplasty was able to establish itself as the leading procedure for the treatment of coronary artery disease. Coronary bypass grafting has maintained its dominance only in patients with diffuse coronary artery disease, diabetes mellitus, left ventricular malfunction and main trunk stenoses. Several comparative studies have underlined the dominance of surgical therapy over angioplasty for the different patient subgroups.

Without doubt, the interventional form of therapy has a special attraction because of its less invasive character which is obvious to the patient. Under the environment of an increasing negative selection of the patient subgroup towards more complex, morphological forms of coronary artery disease, of patients with concomitant diabetes mellitus or left ventricular malfunctions, but also because of the demographic development of patient age, there was natural pressure to develop less invasive surgical techniques. Since sternotomy as a way of accessing the heart is regarded as invasive by many patients and may in fact cause a considerable amount of morbidity, the search for limited accesses to the heart was an initial goal in order to reduce the invasiveness of coronary surgical procedures. Also, the use of the heart-lung machine for coronary surgery was questioned, since with this new kind of operation the heart must not be opened and the use of extracorporeal circulation is basically not required. In this context, a look back towards the first days of coronary bypass grafting is interesting. At the same time as FAVALORO established coronary bypass grafting with the use of the heart-lung machine in Cleveland, a working group from Petersburg headed by KOLESSOV reported on coronary revascularization of the LAD via left lateral thoracotomy on the beating heart without the use of a heart-lung machine in 1967 [16]. After reviewing the subsequent publications, it becomes apparent that some working groups, especially in South America had gathered experience with coronary bypass grafting without the use of the HLM. Particularly BENETTI [1] from Argentina and BUFFOLO [5] from Brazil published reports on the safety and efficiency of coronary bypass surgery without the use of heart-lung machines in a large number of patients. In 1992, PFISTER [22] published an American report on 220 patients in which surgery had been performed without using a heart-lung machine and which were compared to a group of another 220 patients where the HLM was used. There was no statistically significant difference in mortality, but there were advantages concerning the blood loss and post-operative circulation for those patients in which surgery had been performed without a heart-lung machine. In the mid 1990s, these experiences, such as the search for surgical techniques which avoid large complete sternotomy, were brought together. It was again BENETTI [2] and MACK [19] who were the first to describe a video-supported operation technique with a small left antero-lateral thoracotomy for revascularization of the LAD using the left internal mammary artery. This surgical technique has been standardized today under the term MIDCAB surgery. In 1996, the first device was introduced which facilitated the anastomosis of a conduit with the coronary artery on the beating heart by local immobilization [3]. With this, coronary revascularization techniques on the beating heart reached the necessary safety and precision to achieve a quality standard which was reproducible and comparable with conventional strategy on the non-beating heart.

Several working groups, particularly those headed by SUBRA-MANIAN [25], CALAFIORE [6], DIEGELER [7], and TREHAN [26] were able to document the efficiency and safety of this technique in controlled studies in more than 1000 patients each. While MIDCAB surgery combined a limited access to the heart with revascularization without the use of the heart-lung machine, this surgical technique was limited to patients who only required revascularization of the LAD. Parallel to the standardization of MIDCAB surgery, multi-vessel revascularization was developed using special new devices on the beating heart without a heart-lung machine via complete or partial sternotomy. The working group which formed around BORST, JANSEN and GRÜNDEMANN [4, 14] in Utrecht developed a vacuum-supported stabilization system which, on the one hand, stabilized the anastomosis area between the conduit and the coronary artery, but, on the other hand, also helped to expose the coronary vessels in less accessible areas in the lateral, inferior and right lateral regions of the heart. Based on this basic concept, new devices were developed which facilitated local immobilization as well as the exposition of the respective coronary arteries in order to achieve maximum safety, but also offered a comfortable way for surgeons to perform coronary revascularizations on the beating heart. Meanwhile, this technique has also been standardized and the safety and efficiency of this method is supported by numerous publications.

As early as the mid 1990s, strategies were developed to perform heart surgeries endoscopically. The concept of minimally invasive surgery is closely related to videoscopic techniques, as it can be seen in other surgical disciplines. The working group of STEVENS [23] at the Stanford University was the first to develop a catheter system in 1995 which allowed cardioplegic cardiac arrest with extracorporeal circulation without opening the chest. A balloon catheter which was introduced via the femoral artery was used for temporary occlusion of the ascending aorta which allowed cardiac arrest by infusing a cardioplegic solution into the coronary system. This method allowed coronary bypass grafting on the LAD with minimal access to the resting heart on the one hand, but also the use of limited right thoracotomy in the mitral valve in the other hand. This method was also developed and established as a main element of minimally invasive cardiac surgery, especially in mitral valve surgery. In Dresden, GULIELMOS developed a technique where a mini-thoracotomy in the third intercostal space allowed a connection to the heart-lung machine and a limited revascularization of 2 to 3 coronary arteries [13]. The introduction of endoscopic surgical techniques for coronary revascularization includes the difficulty that coronary bypass anastomosis requires very precise microsurgical techniques, which at a certain distance from the target can no longer be performed manually. In order to find a technical solution for this problem, two Californian companies are developing a telemanipulator system which transfers the manual skill of the surgeon to electronically controlled microinstruments.

In May and June 1998, initial operations were performed in parallel in Paris and Leipzig using such a telemanipulator system on the resting heart. A little later, the Leipzig [20] and Dresden [15] working groups also succeeded in performing this operation on the beating heart. This was the first time that coronary bypass grafting on the beating heart was performed endoscopically without opening the chest. Within a few years, we succeeded in technically revolutionizing a surgical technique which had been standardized over 30 years ago. This enormous technical development, but also the further development of a young and innovative generation of surgeons, justifies our hope that coronary bypass grafting will remain a pillar for the treatment of coronary artery disease which with its goal of as little traumatization as possible for the patient and simultaneous highest quality and safety will provide excellent long-term results.

References

1. Benetti FJ, Naselli G, Wood M, Geffner L (1991) Direct myocardial revascularization without extracorporeal circulation. Experience in 700 patients. Chest 100:312–316
2. Benetti FJ, Ballester C (1995) Use of thoracoscopy and a minimal thoracotomy, in mammary-coronary bypass to left anterior descending artery, without extracorporeal circulation. J Cardiovasc Surg 36:159–161
3. Boonstra P, Grandjean J, van Weerd E (1996) Clinical experiences with minimally invasive coronary artery bypass grafting without cardiopulmonary bypass. Programme 10th Annual EACTS, Abstracts:114
4. Borst C, Jansen EW, Tulleken CA et al (1996) Coronary artery bypass grafting without cardiopulmonary bypass and without interruption of native coronary flow using a novel anastomosis site restraining device ("Octopus"). J Am Coll Cardiol 27:1356–1364
5. Buffolo E, Succi AJ, Leao LEV, Gallucci C (1985) Direct myocardial revascularization without cardiopulmonary bypass. J Thorac Cardiovasc Surg 33:26–29
6. Calafiore AM, Di Giammarco G, Teodori G et al (1996) Left anterior descending coronary artery grafting via left anterior small thoracotomy without cardiopulmonary bypass. Ann Thorac Surg 62:1658–1665
7. Diegeler A, Falk V, Matin M, Baltelini R, Walther T, Autschbach R, Mohr FW (1998) Minimally invasive coronary artery bypass grafting. Experience with the MIDCAB approach technique, results and follow-up. Ann Thorac Cardiovasc Surg 66 (3):1022–1025
8. Effler DB, Sones FM, Groves LK, Suarez E (1965) Myocardial revascularisation by Vineberg's internal mammary artery implant: evaluation of postoperative results. J Thorac Cardiovasc Surg 50:527–533
9. Favaloro RG (1968) Saphenous vein autograft replacement of severe segmental coronary artery occlusion: operative technique. Ann Thorac Surg 5:334–339
10. Garrett HE, Dennid EW, DeBakey ME (1973) Aorto-coronary bypass with saphenous vein graft: seven year follow-up. JAMA 223:792–794

11. Gibbon JH Jr (1954) Application of a mechanical heart and lung apparatus to cardiac surgery. Minn Med 37:171–185
12. Grüntzig A (1978) Transluminal dilatation of coronary artery stenosis (letter). Lancet 1:263
13. Gulielmos V, Brandt M, Knaut M, Cichon R, Wagner FM, Kappert U, Schüler S (1999) The Dresden approach for complete multi-vessel revascularization. Ann Thorac Surg 68 (4):1502–1505
14. Jansen EWL (1996) Coronary revascularization on the beating heart using local wall immobilization: the "Octopus" method via limited approach. Programme 10th Annual EACTS, Abstracts: 258
15. Kappert U, Cichon R, Schneider J, Gulielmos V, Tugtekin SM, Matschke K, Schramm I, Schüler S (2000) Closed chest coronary artery surgery on the beating heart with the use of a robotic system. J Thorac Cardiov 120(4):809–811
16. Kolessov VI (1967) Mammary artery-coronary artery anastomosis as a method of treatment for angina pectoris. J Thorac Cardiovasc Surg 54(4):535–544
17. Longmire WP, Cannon JA, Kattus AA (1958) Direct vision coronary endarterectomy for angina pectoris. N Engl J Med 259:993–999
18. Loop FD, Spampinato N, Cheanvechai C, Effler DP (1973) The free internal mammary artery bypass graft. Use of the IMA in the aorta-to-coronary artery position. Ann Thorac Surg 15:50–55
19. Mack M (1996) Minimally invasive thorascopically assisted coronary artery bypass surgery. Programme 10th Annual EACTS 1996, Abstracts: 112
20. Mohr FW, Falk V, Diegeler A, Autschback R (1999) Computer-enhanced coronary artery bypass surgery. J Thorax Surg 117(6): 1212–1214
21. Murray G, Porcheron R, Hilario J et al (1954) Anastomosis of a systemic artery to the coronary. Can Med Assoc J 71:594
22. Pfister AJ, Zaki MS, Garcia JM et al (1992) Coronary artery bypass without cardiopulmonary bypass. J Thorac Surg 54:1085–1091
23. Stevens JN, Burdon TA, Siegel LC et al (1996) Port-access coronary artery bypass with cardioplegic arrest: acute and chronic canine studies. Ann Thorac Surg 62:435–441
24. Sabiston DC, Fauteux JP, Blalock A (1975) An experimental study of the fate of arterial implants in the left ventricular myocardium: with a comparison of similar implants in other organs. Ann Surg 145:927–942

25. Subramanian VA, Sani G, Benetti FJ, Calafiore AM (1995) Minimally invasive coronary bypass surgery: a multicenter report of preliminary clinical experience. Circulation
26. Trehan N, Bapna R et al (1996) Transmyocardial laser revascularization combined with CABG without cardiopulmonary bypass. Programme 10th Annual EACTS 1996; Abstracts: 262

What do we know about OPCAB surgery?

On-pump versus off-pump

I. Friedrich, J. Börgermann

Introduction

Coronary revascularization with extracorporeal circulation (ECC) was established in the 1960s; since then, this technique has evolved into a routine clinical tool. In view of typical mortality rates of 2–5%, the method is generally considered safe. Increasing standardization of the surgical approach and enhanced ECC techniques have led to expanded indications, and subsequently to increasing numbers of elderly patients and patients with multiple morbidities undergoing surgery. These expanded indications confronted us with postoperative complications in patients with complex comorbidities, eventually resulting in higher morbidity and mortality rates and therefore in a higher use of resources. There is a variety of surgical complications which can affect several organ systems. In addition to postoperative hypoperfusion with or without myocardial pump failure, neurological, pulmonary, and renal complications are frequently seen. We should aim at developing therapeutic strategies that minimize surgical trauma without compromising the high safety of the standard approach. In more and more patients, preoperative organ function is already at the brink of decompensation, and the response to an invasive surgical procedure may be enough to threaten this fragile equilibrium. In addition to the surgical procedure, use of the heart-lung machine appears to be a significant factor in the development of postop-

Table 1. Prospective randomized or case matched studies in multivessel off-pump versus on-pump coronary arterial bypass grafting

Study	Year	Pat. no.	Retro-/prospective	Preop. age	Preop. EF	Re-OP	Unstable angina	No. dist. Anast. OPCAB/On-PUMP
Vural et al. [57]	1995	25/25	prosp. random.	47/49	n.s.	0/0	0/0	1.1/1.1
van Dijk et al. [55]	2001	281/281	prosp. random.	62/61	77%/79%	0/0	22%/21%	2.4/2.6 n.s.
Angelini et al. [3]	2002	201/200	prosp. random.	62/62	n.s.	0/0	25%/24%	2.4/2.6 n.s.
Bouchard et al. [12]	1998	40/40	retro.	64/62	?	1.5%/7.5%	72.5% /77.5%	2.8/3.3 $p < 0.01$
Lee et al.[30]	2000	100/100	retro.	66/66	46%/45%	2%/10% $p < 0.05$	?	3.1/3.8 $p < 0.001$
Lancey et al. [29]	2000	76/76	retro.	64.4/64	50%/47%	0/0		2.8/3.7 $p < 0.0001$
Puskas et al. [42]	2001	200/1000	retro.	62/62	?	0/0	?	2.5/3.7 $p < 0.001$
Zamvar et al. [62]	2002	120/247	retro.	63/63	n.s.	0/0	19%/26%	3VD: 2.8/3.0 $p < 0.005$
High-risk subgroups								
Ricci et al. [48]	2000	97/172	retro.	83/82	50%/50%	$p < 0.002$	68%/69%	1.8/3.3 n.s.
Yokoyama [61]	2000	242/483	retro.					3.1/4.0 n.s.

Table 1 (continued)

Study	Stroke	p.o. MI	afib.	Postop. inotropic support	IABP	Transfusion/ bleeding	Incr. myocard.	Enz. renal compl.
Vural et al.	n.s.	0/0	n.s.	4%/25%	4%/0%	*p < 0.001	*p < 0.05	n.s.
van Dijk et al.	n.s.	n.s.	n.s.			*p < 0.01	*p < 0.01	
Angelini et al.	n.s.	n.s.	*p < 0.0001	*p < 0.0001		*p < 0.0001		
Bouchard et al.	n.s.	p = 0.09	n.s.	n.s.	n.s.	n.s.	*p < 0.001	*p = 0.06
Lee et al.	n.s.	n.s.	n.s.			*p < 0.09		*p < 0.04
Lancey et al.	n.s.	n.s.	n.s.			*p < 0.0001		
Puskas et al.						*p < 0.001		
Zamvar et al.			*p < 0.001	*p < 0.002		*p < 0.001		n.s.
High-risk subgroups								
Ricci et al.	*p < 0.005		n.s.		n.s.			n.s.
Yokoyama	n.s.					*p < 0.001		n.s.

Table 1 (continued) A summary of randomized trials and case control studies comparing pre- and postoperative parameters between ON-PUMP and OPCAB surgery

Study	Costs	Postop. Wound Infections	Mortality
Vural et al.	*–21%		n.s.
van Dijk et al.		n.s.	n.s.
Angelini et al.		*p < 0.001	n.s.
Bouchard et al.			n.s.
Lee et al.	*–29%		n.s.
Lancey et al.			n.s.
Puskas et al.	*–15%		n.s.
Zamvar et al.			n.s.
High-risk subgroups			
Ricci et al.			
Yokoyama			

* OPCAB better

erative complications. Retrospective case-control studies indicate that refraining from the use of ECC results in fewer postoperative complications in comparison to the conventional approach. This may be particularly true in high-risk and elderly patients [1, 10, 19, 40, 41, 61]. Currently, there are only two prospective randomized studies on multivessel bypass procedures that allow scientifically valid conclusions regarding the pros and cons of either approach [3, 55]. A potential bias limits the validity of retrospective studies. Extrinsic factors that could affect the results include: 1) selective publication of surgical results, 2) OPCAB patients are a) often younger and b) frequently require only a small number of distal anastomoses, 3) better LV function, 4) possibly more suitable coronary anatomy in the OPCAB group, and 5) different surgical teams performing procedures in different groups; a bias seen in many studies. There is also a large number of published case-control studies that include high-risk patients and compare them with similar groups (Table 1).

Low cardiac output, hypoperfusion

Severely reduced left ventricular pump function is an independent risk factor for bypass surgery. An LV-EF < 30% increases the surgical risk by a factor of 5–10 [60]. The use of ECC and cardioplegic arrest may present an additional, independent risk for these patients. Experimental studies demonstrate that proinflammatory cytokines which are released after reperfusion are cardiac depressants, possibly adding to worsening myocardial function [36]. In addition, the altered geometry of the failing left ventricle as well as coronary artery occlusions or stenoses can lead to inhomogeneous distribution of the cardioplegic solution and therefore to inadequate preservation of the already damaged myocardium [46, 50]. Compared to conventional approaches, recent retrospective studies demonstrate improved postoperative results of OPCAB procedures in patients with reduced LV function [22, 27, 54]. Overall, postoperative inotropic support was required in a smaller percentage of OPCAB cases. The clinical observation of poor tolerance to cardiac manipulation in hearts with restricted LV function does not appear to be primarily related to the degree of LV functional impairment but more to the clinical severity of decompensation (NYHA IV). In patients bordering decompensation who have massively elevated left atrial pressures, the OPCAB approach is often at its limits. IABP support will frequently allow a beating-heart approach only after some period of stabilization [18, 25]. The beating-heart technique is usually applicable for the anterior wall coronary branches, even in cases of highly impaired ventricular function. If ECC support is chosen to bypass the coronary branches of the lateral and posterior wall on the beating heart, the typically needed ECC duration of 10 to 30 min will most likely not result in any substantial problems for the patient. Active bypass graft perfusion prior to constructing the central anastomoses is an elegant technical option when operating on patients with impaired cardiovascular performance. The technique avoids use of the heart-lung machine and guarantees coronary perfusion independent of mean pressure [43, 51], but this approach needs further evaluation. In patients with a high-risk profile and a multitude of comorbid conditions, one should consider hybrid cardiac revascularization: excellent clinical results have been accomplished with this palliative approach that combines minimally invasive surgical revascularization of the easily accessible coronary vessels with PTCA/stenting of the lateral branches in a second session [49]. When developing a therapeutic concept for myocardial revascularization, coronary angiographic data should not be the only focus. What is rather required is an individualized strategy, based on patient-specific selection of therapy options.

Postoperative myocardial infarctions, patency rates

Critics of beating-heart myocardial revascularization are mostly concerned about the quality of the distal anastomoses. One should clearly not underestimate that performing these anastomoses is technically demanding, especially when the heart is hypertrophied and when the coronary arteries of the lateral and posterior wall are small and diffusely diseased. Although the majority of authors did not find differences between postoperative angiographic OPCAB and ON-PUMP graft patency rates – but in fact documented that a smaller amount of Troponin I is released in the OPCAB group [8, 16, 21, 45, 63], KIM et al. observed lower vein bypass patency rates on long-term follow-up. In the OPCAB group, vein bypass patency decreased from 85.6% early after the operation to 67.9% after 1 year, whereas vein bypass patency rates were 86% in patient groups who had undergone ECC. There was no significant difference with respect to arterial graft patency [26]. Omeroglu et al. demonstrated similar results, showing a patency rate of 45.5% for venous bypasses [39]. These findings are probably a reflection of hypercoagulability, as shown by Mariani et al. in a study on OPCAB patients. On the first postoperative day after OPCAB, prothrombin factors 1 and 2 were increased and so was the von Willebrand factor plasma level. According to this study, plasma hypercoagulability was independent of platelet function [31]. Nearly all studies show less postoperative bleeding and therefore lowered transfusion requirements after OPCAB in comparison to conventional revascularization. It is conceivable that this relates to enhanced activation of the coagulation system. The increased bleeding tendency after conventional procedures should not only be seen as a disadvantage, however: an impaired coagulation system resulting from the use of ECC might be a factor protecting venous grafts and increasing their patency rate. Postoperative anticoagulation protocols were empirically adopted from the ON-PUMP approach, and further research is needed to adjust the protocols to

OPCAB-specific requirements. That is the reason for the authors' recommendation to refrain from neutralizing heparin with protamine unless there is excessive bleeding [26].

Myocardial injury

Most studies show that ECC procedures are associated with a higher postoperative release of markers for myocardial ischemia than OPCAB procedures [3, 12, 55]. This finding appears to be independent of the type of cardioplegic solution used (Angelini: warm blood cardioplegia, van Dijk: St. Thomas solution). After OPCAB, there is less mitochondrial and myofibrillar damage, as demonstrated by BENETTI et al. who used myocardial biopsies in patients with acute myocardial infarctions [9]. Pump failure can result from ischemia/reperfusion injury after cardioplegic arrest, especially in hearts with pre-existing myocardial damage. This is corroborated by the observation that postoperative OPCAB patients are hemodynamically more stable and often require less inotropic support [3, 57, 62]. In cases of acute myocardial infarctions, immediate OPCAB surgical revascularization is possibly much more successful than the use of ECC and cardioplegic arrest. VLASSOWV et al. and MOHR et al. report postoperative mortalities of 7.7% and 1.7% in studies on patients with acute myocardial infarctions. It is still speculative as to what extent the published mortality figures of 20–30% in patients with acute myocardial infarctions who underwent revascularization with ECC and cardioplegic arrest are related to the mediator release induced by the no-reflow phenomenon [35, 56].

Pulmonary complications, ARDS

During the early postoperative period, ECC-assisted cardiac surgical procedures are associated with a pronounced reduction of pulmonary function. While this effect tends to be subclinical, 10% of cases develop marked respiratory impairment, including up to 2% who develop full ARDS [38]. With the current use of membrane oxygenators, severe postoperative pulmonary failure combined with pulmonary edema – in the past referred to as "pump lung" – has become a much rarer event. This feared complication was a frequent cause of multiorgan failure which is still associated with a 50% mortality despite all modern intensive care management. The typical initial signs of postoperative respiratory insufficiency include reduced arterial oxygen saturation, reduced dynamic and static compliance, as well as increased pulmonary vascular resistance. Hypoxemia and reduced compliance are caused by changed permeability of the pulmonary vasculature, resulting in an influx of water and plasma proteins into the pulmonary interstitium and eventually into the alveolar space. The subsequent inactivation of surfactant function leads to local areas of atelectasis and increases intrapulmonary shunting [24]. The mechanisms triggering respiratory insufficiency after cardiac surgical procedures are to a great extent identical to those triggering ARDS. Activation of the pro-inflammatory cascades (complement system, cytokines), especially release of TNF-alpha, IL-6, IL-8, and elastase, trigger the permeability change [7]. The resulting pathophysiologic changes are the basis for the development of ARDS. Even when ECC is not used, the overwhelming number of mechanisms possibly responsible for postoperative pulmonary failure simply result from the surgical procedure itself and from anesthesia: dividing the sternum and incising the pleura are important factors. Major abdominal surgical procedures can also cause early postoperative respiratory complications. The main pathogenetic factors relate to patient positioning, artificial ventilation, infusion of plasma expanders, and blood transfusions.

Nearly all patients who undergo general anesthesia including intubation were shown to develop atelectases [14]. In cardiac surgical patients, ECC results in additive or – if comorbid conditions are present – multiplicative damage. Issues specific for ECC are blood contact with a foreign surface, hypothermia, and especially cardiac and pulmonary ischemia and reperfusion [32, 58]. The pathophysiologic changes in cases of pump lung match the inflammatory changes during the development of ARDS. Until now, the OPCAB approach has not been proven to be associated with better pulmonary outcome [52]. Various studies demonstrated diminished release of the pro-inflammatory mediators responsible for the development of SIRS and ARDS, although the clinical importance of these findings remains uncertain [20, 33]. So far, OPCAB has not been proven to be a more preferable approach for patients with pulmonary morbidities. Between patients treated by conventional surgery versus OPCAB, no significant differences have been described with respect to gas exchange and pulmonary function [17].

Renal complications, renal insufficiency requiring dialysis

Extracorporeal circulation appears to result in temporary impairment of renal function, which is clinically unapparent in patients with normal renal function. Patients with normal renal function run a risk of developing perioperative renal failure on the order of magnitude of up to 1% [15]. Until now, the OPCAB approach was not shown to result in a definitive advantage with respect to renal function in patients with normal renal function [23, 53]. The following factors are thought to contribute to the etiology of acute renal failure after cardiac surgical procedures with ECC: non-pulsatile flow, release of inflammatory mediators such as endothelin, elastase, and oxygen-free radicals, as well as hypothermia and renal hypoperfusion.

Duration of ECC correlates with the development of postoperative renal failure closely [15]. Hemoglobin release from damaged blood cells is apparently an additional contributing factor. This risk is of just secondary importance in patients with normal renal function, but in cases of pre-existing renal impairment any additional renal injury during cardiac surgery with ECC presents a considerable factor for increased morbidity and mortality. Compared to patients with normal renal function, patients with preoperatively elevated creatinine levels have a 4-fold risk of developing postoperative renal failure requiring dialysis. The mortality associated with postoperative renal failure requiring dialysis is quoted to be 7–38% [23]. It is questionable whether refraining from use of the heart-lung machine might protect the kidneys of patients with renal impairment and whether the beating-heart approach can prevent additional deterioration of renal function. Ascione et al. found pointers to a protective effect in a group of 253 non-dialysis-dependent patients with renal insufficiency in whom serum creatinine and urea levels increased significantly lower after off-pump revascularization [5]. In a previous publication on patients with normal renal function, the same authors were able to demonstrate that glomerular filtration was much better and tubular reabsorption much less impaired after off-pump procedures [4].

Neurological complications, strokes

One of the most important arguments for the use of OPCAB is the reduced occurrence of neurologic impairment and severe strokes in high-risk patients. Due to the steadily increasing mean age of patients referred for coronary revascularization, the incidence of severe postoperative neurologic deficits is on the rise. While the risk of a stroke after conventional cardiac surgery is quoted to be approximately 1% for the age group of 50–60 years, the incidence doubles with each additional decade of life. Risk factors include the following: previous cerebral insult(s), reduced LV function, unstable angina, and emergency surgery [6, 34, 44]. Treating postoperative strokes is very time consuming and costly. The average stay in intensive care of 1.3 days increases to about 25 days, and the associated mortality is approximately 20%. Of all deaths after cardiac bypass surgery, 18–25% result from perioperative strokes. The late outcome is also much poorer because these patients have a markedly reduced life expectancy. In a study by PUSKAS et al. who included 10 800 patients (including 244 patients who suffered a stroke), 81% of the patients without a stroke, but only 44% of patients with a stroke survived a 5-year postoperative period. There are several triggers for intraoperative strokes. Bowles et al. studied the frequency of microembolic events throughout the various phases of OPCAB and ON-PUMP procedures [13]. Microembolic events were most frequent when the ascending aorta was cannulated, and from initiating ECC until the aorta was unclamped. In the OPCAB group, the cumulative number of microembolic events was 27, but averaged 1766 in the ON-PUMP group (65 times higher). With 70 patients in one and 67 patients in the other group, the rate of strokes (0% vs. 2.9%) was too low to reach statistical significance. Of all microembolic events, 7.6% occurred during aortic cannulation. Not much attention has been paid to partial aortic clamping for constructing proximal anastomoses. According to an autopsy study of cardiac surgical patients by BLAUTH et al., calcified and soft intravascular plaques are strongly correlated with the patients' age [11]. In a study on 102 patients, MURKIN et al. were able to show that the intended aortic cannulation site or site for the proximal anastomoses was changed in 23.5% after intraoperative sonographic assessment of the ascending aorta, thereby reducing the rate of postoperative strokes significantly. The study showed frequent extensive changes inside the aortic lumen which had been undetectable on initial palpatory assessment of the aorta. The authors concluded from their results that epiaortic sonographic evaluation prior to aortic manipulation can significantly lower the risk of stroke [37]. KOBAYASHI et al. favor an "aorta no-touch technique", completely refraining from proximal anastomoses in favor of composite grafts [28]. Future studies with larger patient numbers will demonstrate whether this more involved procedure will bring better overall results.

Non-pulsatile flow with low mean pressures, increased cerebral extravascular fluid [2], and microscopic air bubbles are additional risk factors for cerebral injury under ECC. A comparison of methods in patients without any particular stroke risk reveals inconsistent data. While some authors document a significant reduction of cerebrovascular events, other studies cannot verify such a difference. It is remarkable, however, that no study has ever shown a higher incidence of strokes in the off-pump group. The lowered incidence of postoperative strokes in high-risk patients was documented in several studies. In summary: until now, no studies have shown an advantage for patients with a normal risk for a postoperative stroke. Prospective randomized studies with large patient numbers are still pending.

Costs

Surgical complications represent a significant cost factor for the health care sector. Considering the immediate costs for treating a stroke patient in Germany of 15 000 € and subsequent expenses of 20 000 €, a significant reduction of the risk of just strokes by using the OPCAB approach could save a two-digit amount of million Euros [59]. Model calculations from the international literature are strongly related to the specific national organizational structures and to health care financing issues, so that they can hardly be transferred to other countries and health care systems. Intraoperative costs for a multivessel OPCAB procedure depend on the instruments used. In case of disposables (Axius, Xpose), costs will easily add up to more than what was saved by not having to use ECC tubing sets.

Blower/mister, intravascular shunts, and cell-saver are further items to be tallied. One should not forget that the procedures usually also require more and more experienced surgical and anesthesia personnel. During the critical phases, a perfusionist needs to be on stand-by and is therefore not available for other work. Possible savings for the cardiac surgical departments result from reduced transfusion and dialysis requirements, and a shortened stay in intensive care [47]. The potential savings from a shortened hospital stay secondary to a lower rate of complications are more a benefit to the agency covering the health care costs than to the respective department of cardiac surgery. A general cutback of the insurance carriers' reimbursements for OPCAB procedures should only be implemented after the procedural costs are exactly analyzed and does not appear justifiable at this time.

Summary

OPCAB has become a safe alternative to conventional revascularization. Prospective randomized studies could already demonstrate clinical advantages for patients with average risk profiles. Future prospective randomized studies in high-risk patients will delineate benefits and potential risks.

References

1. Akpinar B, Guden M, Sanisoglu I, Sagbas E, Caynak B, Bayramoglu Z et al (2001) Does off-pump coronary artery bypass surgery reduce mortality in high risk patients? Heart Surg Forum 4(3):231–236
2. Anderson RE, Li TQ, Hindmarsh T, Settergren G, Vaage J (1999) Increased extracellular brain water after coronary artery bypass

grafting is avoided by off-pump surgery. J Cardiothorac Vasc Anesth 13(6):698–702

3. Angelini GD, Taylor FC, Reeves BC, Ascione R (2002) Early and midterm outcome after off-pump and on-pump surgery in Beating Heart Against Cardioplegic Arrest Studies (BHACAS 1 and 2): a pooled analysis of two randomised controlled trials. Lancet 359(9313):1194–1199

4. Ascione R, Lloyd CT, Underwood MJ, Gomes WJ, Angelini GD (1999) On-pump versus off-pump coronary revascularization: evaluation of renal function. Ann Thorac Surg 68(2):493–498

5. Ascione R, Nason G, Al-Ruzzeh S, Ko C, Ciulli F, Angelini GD (2001) Coronary revascularization with or without cardiopulmonary bypass in patients with preoperative nondialysis-dependent renal insufficiency. Ann Thorac Surg 72(6):2020–2025

6. Ascione R, Reeves BC, Chamberlain MH, Ghosh AK, Lim KH, Angelini GD (2002) Predictors of stroke in the modern era of coronary artery bypass grafting: a case control study. Ann Thorac Surg 74(2):474–480

7. Asimakopoulos G, Smith PL, Ratnatunga CP, Taylor KM (1999) Lung injury and acute respiratory distress syndrome after cardiopulmonary bypass. Ann Thorac Surg 68(3):1107–1115

8. Bedi HS, Suri A, Kalkat MS, Sengar BS, Mahajan V, Chawla R et al (2000) Global myocardial revascularization without cardiopulmonary bypass using innovative techniques for myocardial stabilization and perfusion. Ann Thorac Surg 69(1):156–164

9. Benetti FJ, Mariani MA, Ballester C (1996) Direct coronary surgery without cardiopulmonary bypass in acute myocardial infarction. J Cardiovasc Surg (Torino) 37(4):391–395

10. Bittner HB, Savitt MA (2002) Off-pump coronary artery bypass grafting decreases morbidity and mortality in a selected group of high-risk patients. Ann Thorac Surg 74(1):115–118

11. Blauth CI, Cosgrove DM, Webb BW, Ratliff NB, Boylan M, Piedmonte MR et al (1992) Atheroembolism from the ascending aorta. An emerging problem in cardiac surgery. J Thorac Cardiovasc Surg 103(6):1104–111; discussion 11–12.

12. Bouchard D, Cartier R (1998) Off-pump revascularization of multivessel coronary artery disease has a decreased myocardial infarction rate. Eur J Cardiothorac Surg 14 (Suppl 1):S20–S24

13. Bowles BJ, Lee JD, Dang CR, Taoka SN, Johnson EW, Lau EM et al (2001) Coronary artery bypass performed without the use of car-

diopulmonary bypass is associated with reduced cerebral micro-emboli and improved clinical results. Chest 119(1):25–30

14. Brismar B, Hedenstierna G, Lundquist H, Strandberg A, Svensson L, Tokics L (1985) Pulmonary densities during anesthesia with muscular relaxation – a proposal of atelectasis. Anesthesiology 62(4):422–428

15. Chertow GM, Lazarus JM, Christiansen CL, Cook EF, Hammermeister KE, Grover F et al (1997) Preoperative renal risk stratification. Circulation 95(4):878–884

16. Contini M, Di Mauro M, Vitolla G, Mazzei V, Iaco AL, Cirmeni S et al (2000) Off-pump myocardial revascularization using arterial conduits without cardiopulmonary bypass. J Card Surg 15(4):251–255

17. Cox CM, Ascione R, Cohen AM, Davies IM, Ryder IG, Angelini GD (2000) Effect of cardiopulmonary bypass on pulmonary gas exchange: a prospective randomized study. Ann Thorac Surg 69(1):140–145

18. Craver JM, Murrah CP (2001) Elective intraaortic balloon counterpulsation for high-risk off-pump coronary artery bypass operations. Ann Thorac Surg 71(4):1220–1223

19. D'Ancona G, Karamanoukian H, Kawaguchi AT, Ricci M, Salerno TA, Bergsland J (2001) Myocardial revascularization of the beating heart in high-risk patients. J Card Surg 16(2):132–139

20. Diegeler A, Doll N, Rauch T, Haberer D, Walther T, Falk V et al (2000) Humoral immune response during coronary artery bypass grafting: a comparison of limited approach, "off-pump" technique, and conventional cardiopulmonary bypass. Circulation 102(19 Suppl 3):III95–100

21. Diegeler A, Matin M, Falk V, Battellini R, Walther T, Autschbach R et al (1999) Coronary bypass grafting without cardiopulmonary bypass – technical considerations, clinical results, and follow-up. Thorac Cardiovasc Surg 47(1):14–18

22. Eryilmaz S, Corapcioglu T, Eren NT, Yazicioglu L, Kaya K, Akalin H (2002) Off-pump coronary artery bypass surgery in the left ventricular dysfunction. Eur J Cardiothorac Surg 21(1):36–40

23. Gamoso MG, Phillips-Bute B, Landolfo KP, Newman MF, Stafford-Smith M (2000) Off-pump versus on-pump coronary artery bypass surgery and postoperative renal dysfunction. Anesth Analg 91(5):1080–1084

24. Gunther A, Siebert C, Schmidt R, Ziegler S, Grimminger F, Yabut M et al (1996) Surfactant alterations in severe pneumonia, acute respiratory distress syndrome, and cardiogenic lung edema. Am J Respir Crit Care Med 153(1):176–184

25. Kim KB, Lim C, Ahn H, Yang JK (2001) Intraaortic balloon pump therapy facilitates posterior vessel off-pump coronary artery by-pass grafting in high-risk patients. Ann Thorac Surg 71(6):1964–1968

26. Kim KB, Lim C, Lee C, Chae IH, Oh BH, Lee MM et al (2001) Off-pump coronary artery bypass may decrease the patency of saphenous vein grafts. Ann Thorac Surg 72(3):S1033–S1037

27. Kirali K, Rabus MB, Yakut N, Toker ME, Erdogan HB, Balkanay M et al (2002) Early- and long-term comparison of the on- and off-pump bypass surgery in patients with left ventricular dysfunction. Heart Surg Forum 5(2):177–181

28. Kobayashi J, Sasako Y, Bando K, Niwaya K, Tagusari O, Nakajima H et al (2002) Multiple off-pump coronary revascularization with "Aorta No-Touch" technique using composite and sequential methods. Heart Surg Forum 5(2):114–118

29. Lancey RA, Soller BR, Van der Salm TJ (2000) Off-pump versus on-pump coronary artery bypass surgery: a case-matched comparison of clinical outcomes and costs. Heart Surg Forum 3(4):277–281

30. Lee JH, Abdelhady K, Capdeville M (2000) Clinical outcomes and resource usage in 100 consecutive patients after off-pump coronary bypass procedures. Surgery 128(4):548–555

31. Mariani MA, Gu YJ, Boonstra PW, Grandjean JG, van Oeveren W, Ebels T (1999) Procoagulant activity after off-pump coronary operation: is the current anticoagulation adequate? Ann Thorac Surg 67(5):1370–1375

32. Massoudy P, Zahler S, Becker BF, Braun SL, Barankay A, Meisner H (2001) Evidence for inflammatory responses of the lungs during coronary artery bypass grafting with cardiopulmonary bypass. Chest 119(1):31–36

33. Matata BM, Sosnowski AW, Galinanes M (2000) Off-pump bypass graft operation significantly reduces oxidative stress and inflammation. Ann Thorac Surg 69(3):785–791

34. McKhann GM, Goldsborough MA, Borowicz LM Jr, Mellits ED, Brookmeyer R, Quaskey SA et al (1997) Predictors of stroke risk in coronary artery bypass patients. Ann Thorac Surg 63(2):516–521

35. Mohr R, Moshkovitch Y, Shapira I, Amir G, Hod H, Gurevitch J (1999) Coronary artery bypass without cardiopulmonary bypass for patients with acute myocardial infarction. J Thorac Cardiovasc Surg 118(1):50–56

36. Muller-Werdan U, Schumann H, Fuchs R, Reithmann C, Loppnow H, Koch S et al (1997) Tumor necrosis factor alpha (TNF alpha) is cardiodepressant in pathophysiologically relevant concentrations without inducing inducible nitric oxide-(NO)-synthase (iNOS) or triggering serious cytotoxicity. J Mol Cell Cardiol 29(11):2915–2923

37. Murkin JM (2000) Neurological outcomes after OPCAB: how much better is it? Heart Surg Forum 3(3):207–210

38. Ng CS, Wan S, Yim AP, Arifi AA (2002) Pulmonary dysfunction after cardiac surgery. Chest 121(4):1269–1277

39. Omeroglu SN, Kirali K, Guler M, Toker ME, Ipek G, Isik O et al (2000) Midterm angiographic assessment of coronary artery bypass grafting without cardiopulmonary bypass. Ann Thorac Surg 70(3):844–849; discussion 50

40. Perrault LP, Menasche P, Peynet J, Faris B, Bel A, de Chaumaray T et al (1997) On-pump, beating-heart coronary artery operations in high-risk patients: an acceptable trade-off? Ann Thorac Surg 64(5): 1368–1373

41. Pompilio G, Zanobini M, Polvani G, Alamanni F, Bignoli P (2001) Efficacy of off-pump coronary artery bypass grafting in high-risk patients. Ann Thorac Surg 71(5):1750–1751

42. Puskas JD, Thourani VH, Marshall JJ, Dempsey SJ, Steiner MA, Sammons BH et al (2001) Clinical outcomes, angiographic patency, and resource utilization in 200 consecutive off-pump coronary bypass patients. Ann Thorac Surg 71(5):1477–1483; discussion 83–84

43. Puskas JD, Thourani VH, Vinten-Johansen J, Guyton RA (2001) Active perfusion of coronary grafts facilitates complex off-pump coronary artery bypass surgery. Heart Surg Forum 4(1):65–68

44. Puskas JD, Winston AD, Wright CE, Gott JP, Brown WM 3rd, Craver JM et al (2000) Stroke after coronary artery operation: incidence, correlates, outcome, and cost. Ann Thorac Surg 69(4):1053–1056

45. Puskas JD, Wright CE, Ronson RS, Brown WM, 3rd, Gott JP, Guyton RA (1998) Off-pump multivessel coronary bypass via sternotomy is safe and effective. Ann Thorac Surg 66(3):1068–1072

46. Quintilio C, Voci P, Bilotta F, Luzi G, Chiarotti F, Acconcia MC et al (1995) Risk factors of incomplete distribution of cardioplegic

solution during coronary artery grafting. J Thorac Cardiovasc Surg 109(3):439–447

47. Reichenspurner H, Boehm D, Detter C, Schiller W, Reichart B (1999) Economic evaluation of different minimally invasive procedures for the treatment of coronary artery disease. Eur J Cardiothorac Surg 16 (Suppl 2):76–79

48. Ricci M, Karamanoukian HL, Abraham R, Von Fricken K, D'Ancona G, Choi S et al (2000) Stroke in octogenarians undergoing coronary artery surgery with and without cardiopulmonary bypass. Ann Thorac Surg (5):1471–1475

49. Riess FC, Bader R, Kremer P, Kuhn C, Kormann J, Mathey D et al (2002) Coronary hybrid revascularization from January 1997 to January 2001: a clinical follow-up. Ann Thorac Surg 73(6):1849–1855

50. Stamou SC, Dangas G, Dullum MK, Pfister AJ, Boyce SW, Bafi AS et al (2000) Beating heart surgery in octogenarians: perioperative outcome and comparison with younger age groups. Ann Thorac Surg 69(4):1140–1145

51. Steele M, Palmer-Steele C (2000) Perfusion technique for perfusion-assisted direct coronary artery bypass (PADCAB). J Extra Corpor Technol 32(3):158–161

52. Taggart DP (2000) Respiratory dysfunction after cardiac surgery: effects of avoiding cardiopulmonary bypass and the use of bilateral internal mammary arteries. Eur J Cardiothorac Surg 18(1):31–37

53. Tang AT, Knott J, Nanson J, Hsu J, Haw MP, Ohri SK (2002) A prospective randomized study to evaluate the renoprotective action of beating heart coronary surgery in low risk patients. Eur J Cardiothorac Surg 22(1):118–123

54. Tugtekin SM, Gulielmos V, Cichon R, Kappert U, Matschke K, Knaut M et al (2000) Off-pump surgery for anterior vessels in patients with severe dysfunction of the left ventricle. Ann Thorac Surg 0(3):1034–1036

55. van Dijk D, Nierich AP, Jansen EW, Nathoe HM, Suyker WJ, Diephuis JC et al (2001) Early outcome after off-pump versus on-pump coronary bypass surgery: results from a randomized study. Circulation 104(15):1761–1766

56. Vlassov GP, Deyneka CS, Travine NO, Timerbaev VH, Ermolov AS (2001) Acute myocardial infarction: OPCAB is an alternative approach for treatment. Heart Surg Forum 4(2):147–150

57. Vural KM, Tasdemir O, Karagoz H, Emir M, Tarcan O, Bayazit K (1995) Comparison of the early results of coronary artery bypass grafting with and without extracorporeal circulation. Thorac Cardiovasc Surg 43(6):320–325

58. Wan S, DeSmet JM, Barvais L, Goldstein M, Vincent JL, LeClerc JL (1996) Myocardium is a major source of proinflammatory cytokines in patients undergoing cardiopulmonary bypass. J Thorac Cardiovasc Surg 112(3):806–811

59. Weimar C, Stausberg J, Kraywinkel K, Wagner M, Busse O, Haberl RL et al (2002) [Diagnosis related groups in stroke treatment. An analysis from the stroke data bank of the German Stroke Foundation]. Dtsch Med Wochenschr 127(31/32):1627–1632

60. Yau TM, Fedak PW, Weisel RD, Teng C, Ivanov J (1999) Predictors of operative risk for coronary bypass operations in patients with left ventricular dysfunction. J Thorac Cardiovasc Surg 118(6): 1006–1013

61. Yokoyama T, Baumgartner FJ, Gheissari A, Capouya ER, Panagiotides GP, Declusin RJ (2000) Off-pump versus on-pump coronary bypass in high-risk subgroups. Ann Thorac Surg 70(5):1546–1550

62. Zamvar VY, Khan NU, Madhavan A, Nihal Kulatilake NK, Butchart EG (2002) Clinical outcomes in coronary artery bypass graft surgery: comparison of off-pump and on-pump techniques. Heart Surg Forum 5(2):109–113

63. Zehr KJ, Handa N, Bonilla LF, Abel MD, Holmes DR, Jr (2000) Pitfalls and results of immediate angiography after off-pump coronary artery bypass grafting. Heart Surg Forum 3(4):293–299

Systemic inflammatory response after cardiac surgery: Is extracorporeal circulation the main culprit?

J. Börgermann, I. Friedrich

Introduction

Cardiac surgery with extracorporeal circulation (ECC) is associated with a systemic inflammatory response [28, 53]. Kirklin and coworkers described this phenomenon as early as 1981 and coined the term *postperfusion syndrome* [13]. In the majority of cases, the organism can fully compensate for this *systemic inflammatory response syndrome* (SIRS). But any postoperative exacerbation will increase morbidity and mortality. Surgical trauma, ischemia/reperfusion, endotoxinemia, and cellular activation induced by shear-stress and by the foreign-surfaces of the heart-lung machine are pathophysiological mechanisms that activate the systemic inflammatory response (Fig. 1).

One of the proposed advantages of *off-pump coronary bypass surgery* (OPCAB) is that some of these triggers for inflammation are avoided, especially global ischemia/reperfusion and extracorporeal circulation. But clinical signs of a systemic inflammatory response can also be observed after off-pump operations, i.e., fever, decreased vascular resistance, and hypotension. In parallel, inflammatory markers increase postoperatively, e.g., C-reactive protein, lipopolysaccharide binding protein (LBP), and procalcitonin [4, 21]. The following literature review compares the SIRS-related mediator systems in on-pump versus off-pump cardiac surgery.

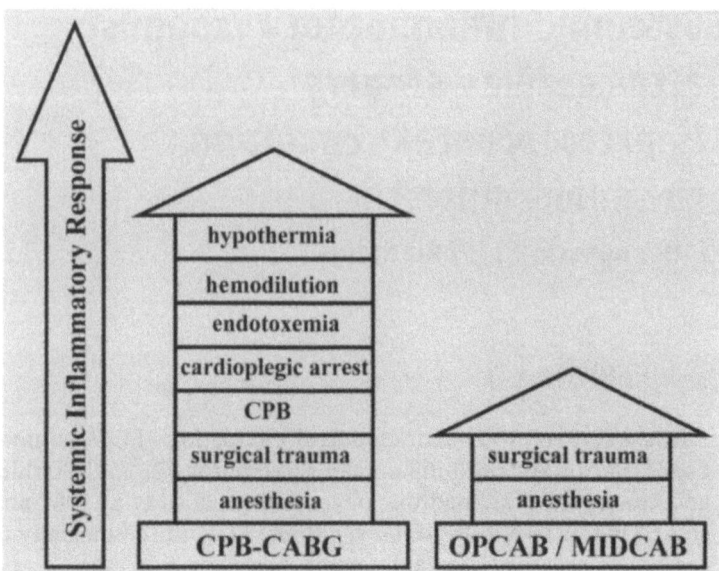

Fig. 1. Pathophysiological "building blocks" that contribute to the systemic inflammatory response syndrome in on-pump (CPB-CABG) and off-pump coronary surgery (OPCAB and MIDCAB). *CPB* cardiopulmonary bypass; *CPB-CABG* cardiopulmonary bypass/coronary artery bypass grafting; *OPCAB* off-pump coronary artery bypass grafting; *MIDCAB* minimal invasive direct coronary artery bypass grafting

Complement activation

The complement system is a cascade system, and the cascade can be activated via the classical or the alternate pathway. The anaphylatoxins C3a and C5a are split products of the complement cascade. They are potent leukocyte and platelet activators, raise vascular permeability, cause vasodilatation, and the release of histamine, oxygen-free radicals, and lysosomal enzymes. The terminal complement complex C5b-9 is also called the *membrane attack* complex. It activates leucocytes and endothelial cells just like the anaphylatoxins C3a and C5a do. Studies on patients who underwent surgery with extracorporeal circulation showed that postoperatively elevated C3a levels are correlated with higher complication rates [31] and prolonged artificial ventilation [38]. Seghaye and coworkers observed in children who later developed MOF (multi-organ failure) that the C3 conversion rate was increased and prolonged [46].

Since activation of the alternate pathway is primarily attributed to blood contacting the foreign surfaces inside the heart-lung machine, it is thought that the complement system does not play any or just a minor role in the development of SIRS after off-pump surgery. One hour postoperatively, Ascione found significantly higher C3a and C5a levels in the on-pump group [2]. During the further course (4–24 hours postoperatively), there were no longer any significant differences between the two groups. Strüber and coworkers studied MIDCAB patients (off-pump via anterior thoracotomy) in comparison to patients treated with conventional on-pump CABG surgery. The authors demonstrated both significantly elevated C3a levels and reduced activity of the C1 esterase inhibitor in the on-pump group [47]. No changes were seen in the MIDCAB group. Gu was able to show that the operative trauma activates the complement system *per se*. In his prospective study, he reported elevated C3a levels in MIDCAB and OPCAB patients whose surgical procedure had included a median sternotomy [26]. Compared to the on-pump groups, C3a peak levels were lower by a factor of 5–10. These studies show, on the one hand, that extracorporeal circulation is the main activator of the complement system. On the other hand, other pathophysiological mechanisms, such as surgical trauma, appear to contribute to the activation of the complement cascade as well. It is therefore likely that the complement system does in fact play a role in the inflammatory response seen in association with off-pump surgery.

▌ Leukocyte and endothelial cell activation

Leukocyte and endothelial cell activation are important players in the pathophysiological sequence that eventually causes organ damage via the inflammatory response. This process involves binding of activated leukocytes to endothelial adhesion molecules, e.g., to the intracellular molecule (ICAM)-1, via specific ligands, e.g., CD11b/CD18 (also known as Mac-1) on peripheral blood mononuclear cells (PBMNC). The now attached leukocytes migrate through the endothelial layer to the target organ *(margination)*, where they release proteases, oxygen radicals, and leukotrienes that injure the organ's parenchyma. Adhesion molecules are induced by cytokines (TNFα, IL-1β, IL-8), leukotrienes (LTB$_4$), platelet activating factor (PAF), lipopolysaccharides and complement (C3a, C5a).

Activation of leukocytes and expression of adhesion molecules have been frequently demonstrated after procedures with ECC, both experimentally [18] and clinically [3, 23, 29, 43]. Results of animal experiments indicate that the interaction between leukocytes and endothelium does play a major role in perioperative lung [24, 25] and myocardial ischemia/reperfusion injury [57].

Several authors report rapidly increasing perioperative leukocyte counts, both in the off-pump as well as in the on-pump groups [2, 7, 26]. Ascione describes that the groups were significantly different in this respect, a finding not corroborated by DIEGELER et al. [17]. This working group finds comparable increases of the total leukocyte count and the granulocyte fraction in the ECC-CABG, OPCAB, and MIDCAB group. The authors report a delayed increase in the off-pump groups. Beyond these changed cell counts, increased levels of leukocyte elastase [2, 36] and bactericidal permeability increasing protein (BPI) [21] are reported after off-pump surgical procedures. In view of the observed kinetics of these serum markers of leukocyte activation, it is evident that the differences between groups are greatest during the immediate postoperative phase (1–4 h) and pretty much disappear during the subsequent course. This is reflected in the cell kinetics described by DIEGELER et al.

The role of leukocyte surface molecules in off-pump surgery has not been investigated. Current results need to be interpreted as such that leukocyte activation is initially accelerated under ECC, but primarily determined by the surgical trauma *per se*.

In addition to leukocyte activation, endothelial expression of adhesion molecules plays a key role in the inflammatory response. Circulating soluble serum adhesion molecules were measured during cardiac surgical procedures with and without ECC. The results are inconsistent. While BOLDT et al. report a reduction of the soluble endothelial leukocyte adhesion molecules (ELAM)-1, ICAM-1, and vascular adhesion molecule (VCAM)-1 in children under ECC and did not observe any changes in adults [5], other authors describe a significant increase of ICAM-1 24 hours after ECC [23, 37]. Among the soluble adhesion molecules, E-selectin, P-selectin, and ICAM-1 were measured in off-pump cases. In a prospective randomized study, Matata found in the on-pump group that E-selectin increased significantly 8 hours postoperatively, but did not increase in the off-pump population [36]. Using immunohistochemical methods, WILDHIRT elegantly demonstrated that the endomyocardial expression of P-selectin and ICAM-1 is elevated in the on-pump group and that it is accompanied by increased expression of tumor necrosis factor-a (TNFa) [55]. Whether this increased expression is specific for cardioplegic arrest, for ECC, or for both, could not be determined with this particular study design. These data seem to confirm, however, that off-pump surgery is not associated with any significant cellular activation.

▌ Cytokine release

Cytokines are peptides or glycoproteins. They provide bi-directional communication between various groups of leukocytes and also between leukocytes and parenchymal cells. They bind to specific receptors and their mechanism of action is either autocrine or paracrine. Cytokines are important regulators of the non-specific and the antigen-specific immune response. Numerous studies have been published comparing the release of pro- and anti-inflammatory cytokines in on-pump and off-pump surgery.

▌ **Tumor necrosis factor-α (TNFα)** is a proinflammatory cytokine produced by neutrophils, monocytes, and endothelial cells. TNFα activates leukocytes and enhances the expression of adhesion molecules on endothelial cells. TNFα therefore assumes a key position in both the local and the systemic inflammatory response. TNFα affects hemostasis. While TNFα increases thrombin formation, it inhibits fibrinolysis. TNFα additionally induces a hyperdynamic circulatory response characterized by tachycardia and loss of peripheral vascular resistance. It also has negative inotropic effects. Published studies report consistently higher TNFα as well as TNF receptor levels (TNF-Rp55 and TNF-Rp75) in patients undergoing operations with ECC [16, 36, 44, 47]. Studies conducted by WAN et al. allow the conclusion that TNFα release is primarily the result of ischemia/reperfusion injury and not due to ECC *per se*. WAN was able to show that considerable amounts of TNFα are primarily released by the myocardium after reperfusion [49]. TNFα kinetics and the kinetics of its receptors, both of which rise sharply after reperfusion, support this conclusion. It has also been demonstrated that the production of TNFα in blood decreases after ECC [6, 39].

▌ **Interleukin (IL)-6** has pro- and anti-inflammatory properties. It is important for the immune response and acute phase reaction. IL-6 affects the hypothalamo-pituitary axis to the effect of an increased cortisol release. But it also inhibits the production of other proinflammatory cytokines such as TNFα and IL-1β. All published studies show a peri- or postoperative release in both off-pump and on-pump procedures. Differences between the groups are not consistent, however. Whereas DIEGELER and Wan find either no or only very small differences between the on-pump and off-pump groups [16, 50], STRÜBER, SCHULZE and FRANSEN report significant differences until 8 hours postoperatively [21, 44, 47]. GULIELMOS found no relationship between the use of ECC and IL-6 release [27]. Such inconsistencies of the published data on IL-6 indicate that release of this pleiotropic cytokine is not only determined by ECC and ischemia, but also by the extent of surgical trauma; a fact further corroborated by the study published by GU [26].

▌ Interleukin (IL)-8 has chemotactic properties and is responsible for recruiting neutrophils at the site of the inflammatory response. IL-8 activates leukocytes and endothelial cells and is also produced by these cells. Increased IL-8 mRNA expression was shown in animal experiments after reperfusion [32] and in human myocardium after ECC [8]. One can therefore assume that IL-8 contributes to myocardial ischemia/reperfusion injury. As early as 1993, KAWAMURA was able to show a correlation between ischemic time, myocardial injury, and IL-8 in patients undergoing operations with ECC [30]. WAN confirms these results. He reports significant IL-8 release in the on-pump, but not in the off-pump group, and this release correlates with postoperative troponin-I levels [50]. Studies by STRÜBER and DIEGELER also show significantly higher IL-8 levels in the on-pump groups [16, 47]. So IL-8 acts similar to TNFα and is primarily associated with the ischemic event.

▌ Interleukin (IL)-10 is an anti-inflammatory cytokine. It suppresses the synthesis of proinflammatory cytokines *in vitro* and *in vivo* [14, 42]. In a recently published study, YANG was able to demonstrate that endogenously produced IL-10 limits myocardial reperfusion injury [56]. IL-10 release after operations with ECC was demonstrated in several studies [45, 51, 52]. Comparing off-pump versus on-pump procedures, WAN and DIEGELER found significantly elevated IL-10 levels after reperfusion in the on-pump groups, whereas no significant IL-10 release was found in the off-pump groups [16, 50]. Especially the release kinetics allows the conclusion that ischemia/reperfusion stimulates the production of IL-10. Experimental research lends further support to the important role of IL-10 in limiting the injury secondary to inflammation.

Vascular endothelial growth factor and endothelial progenitor cells

Vascular endothelial growth factor (VEGF) is a protein that stimulates angioneogenesis and neovascularization, inhibits intimal hyperplasia and exhibits cardioprotective properties [40]. Hypoxia and vascular trauma stimulate the release of this angiogenetic factor. Endothelial progenitor cells (EPC) are endothelial precursor cells that are mobilized from the bone marrow to promote vascular healing. Recent studies demonstrated that serum VEGF levels increase markedly after operations with ECC, and that there is also a nearly 50-fold increase of EPCs in peripheral blood [22]. BURTON and coauthors were able to demonstrate that postoperatively, serum VEGF increases significantly in both on-pump as well as off-pump cardiac surgical patients. In this study, measured concentrations were comparable between both groups [9]. *In vitro* VEGF release from neonatal rat myocardiocytes could be stimulated by hypoxia. How EPCs relate to OPCAB procedures remains unknown. VEGF release is probably important for graft endothelialization in off-pump and on-pump coronary artery surgery.

Immune cell function

After procedures with ECC, both cellular and humoral immune responses are impaired. As early as 1992, Nguyen was able to show that immediately after ECC, the ratio of CD8+ suppressor/cytotoxic T cells to CD4+ helper/inducer T cells shifts in favor of the CD8+ cells. In addition, the activity of cytotoxic T lymphocytes and natural killer cells remains impaired until the third postoperative day [41]. The synthesis of both essential cytokines [6, 35, 39] and HLA-DR expression on monocytes is decreased after ECC [20]. Both effects lead to dysregulation of the host defense mechanisms. Studies showed that *in vivo* release of cytokine-inhibitory activities [6], and also foreign surfaces and shear stress in the extracorporeal circuit [15] cause this kind of dysregulation of the cell-mediated immune response.

DIEGELER examined T-lymphocyte subsets in patients who had undergone OPCAB, MIDCAB, or conventional cardiac surgical procedures with ECC. He found that four hours postoperatively the number of CD4+ helper/inducer T cells was reduced in all three groups, so that the CD4+/CD8+ ratio decreased [17]. There were no significant differences between the groups. These data could be interpreted as such that the surgical trauma *per se* is the main cause of immune dysregulation. How other immune cell functions, such as their ability to synthesize cytokines or HLA-DR expression on monocytes, respond to off-pump coronary artery bypass surgery, remains to be investigated, however. It is mandatory to assess immune cell function in larger patient populations undergoing off-pump surgery in order to estimate how prone these patients are to infections and to delayed wound healing in comparison to patients who undergo surgery with ECC support.

Oxidative stress

Activated leukocytes can release oxygen-free radicals, and so can ischemic tissues upon reperfusion. Oxygen-free radicals impair the function of antiproteases and therefore the inhibition of elastase. It has been shown that free radicals are produced and released in on-pump procedures [12].

Various studies seem to indicate that oxidative stress is significantly reduced in off-pump coronary surgery. After ECC, hydroperoxides, protein carbonyls, and nitrotyrosine were found to be significantly increased [36]. In the off-pump group, these metabolites were not affected. WILDHIRT investigated the role of malondialdehyde (MDA), which is a product of lipid peroxidation, and can be found in plasma and myocardial tissue. He demonstrated that both plasma as well myocardial MDA increased in the on-pump, but not in the off-pump group [54]. The above studies did not clarify, however, whether ECC or ischemia/reperfusion injury, or a combination of both are the causes of oxidative stress.

Coagulation

Foreign surfaces inside the ECC circuit and exposed collagen from tissue injury directly activate platelets and factor XII. Activated platelets release thromboxane A2 which causes them to aggregate. Factor XIIa and XIIf activate the coagulation and complement system as well as leukocytes and endothelial cells. But ECC also leads to increased fibrinolysis. Fibrin split products inhibit aggregation and fibrin polymerization (for a review see [10, 19]). Coagulation and fibrinolysis are closely and mutually interacting with the inflammatory cascade. The combination of these effects leads to capillary injury with subsequent fluid extravasation and impaired homeostasis.

Homeostasis remains intact after off-pump coronary surgery. This results in less hemorrhage and decreased transfusion requirements compared to on-pump procedures, a fact that has been proven in randomized studies [1, 48]. Preserved homeostasis, however, will also promote a procoagulant state with a potentially higher risk of thrombotic events and early bypass occlusion. MARIANI demonstrated in a study on OPCAB and MIDCAB patients that procoagulant activity is increased during the initial 24 hours after off-pump coronary surgery [34]. Data obtained by CASATI show that both antithrombin and fibrinogen are consumed after on-pump procedures, but also after off-pump cases. In operations performed with ECC support, this is accompanied by dropping platelet counts, plasminogen activation, and increased D-dimer formation [11]. These factors counteract the postoperatively increased procoagulant activity, thereby probably protecting graft and anastomotic patency.

A more aggressive anticoagulation regimen should therefore be considered in off-pump procedures. We would like to emphasize in this context that it is safe to administer acetyl salicylic acid (ASA) early after coronary bypass surgery. ASA is associated with both reduced mortality figures and a lower incidence of ischemic complications [33].

▍ Summary

The results of all published studies comparing the systemic inflammatory response syndrome as it relates to off-pump versus on-pump surgery can be summarized by stating that the differences are primarily quantitative in nature, not qualitative. In other words, activation of the various mediator systems (complement, coagulation, cytokines) and cells (leukocytes, platelets, endothelial cells) does not depend on the surgical approach, but the patterns and extent of activation vary. Available reports are inconclusive for a *resumé* on SIRS in off-pump surgery. Studies analyzing the relationship between mediator systems and the clinical course (end-organ dysfunction) in large numbers of patients who undergo coronary bypass surgery, will demonstrate to what extent off-pump surgery is more than just theoretically superior to on-pump surgery.

References

1. Angelini GD, Taylor FC, Reeves BC, Ascione R (2002) Early and midterm outcome after off-pump and on-pump surgery in Beating Heart Against Cardioplegic Arrest Studies (BHACAS 1 and 2): a pooled analysis of two randomised controlled trials. Lancet 359: 1194–1199
2. Ascione R, Lloyd CT, Underwood MJ, Lotto AA, Pitsis AA, Angelini GD (2000) Inflammatory response after coronary revascularization with or without cardiopulmonary bypass. Ann Thorac Surg 69:1198–1204
3. Asimakopoulos G, Taylor KM (1998) Effects of cardiopulmonary bypass on leukocyte and endothelial adhesion molecules. Ann Thorac Surg 66:2135–2144
4. Bitkover CY, Hansson LO, Valen G, Vaage J (2000) Effects of cardiac surgery on some clinically used inflammation markers and procalcitonin. Scand Cardiovasc J 34:307–314
5. Boldt J, Osmer C, Linke LC, Dapper F, Hempelmann G (1995) Circulating adhesion molecules in pediatric cardiac surgery. Anesth Analg 81:1129–1135
6. Börgermann J, Friedrich I, Flohe S et al (2002) Tumor necrosis factor-α production in whole blood after cardiopulmonary bypass: Downregulation caused by circulating cytokine-inhibitory activities. J Thorac Cardiovasc Surg 124:608–617
7. Brasil LA, Gomes WJ, Salomao R, Buffolo E (1998) Inflammatory response after myocardial revascularization with or without cardiopulmonary bypass. Ann Thorac Surg 66:56–59
8. Burns SA, Newburger JW, Xiao M, Mayer JE, Jr., Walsh AZ, Neufeld EJ (1995) Induction of interleukin-8 messenger RNA in heart and skeletal muscle during pediatric cardiopulmonary bypass. Circulation 92:II315–321
9. Burton PB, Owen VJ, Hafizi S et al (2000) Vascular endothelial growth factor release following coronary artery bypass surgery: extracorporeal circulation versus 'beating heart' surgery. Eur Heart J 21:1708–1713

10. Butler J, Rocker GM, Westaby S (1993) Inflammatory response to cardiopulmonary bypass. Ann Thorac Surg 55: 552–559
11. Casati V, Gerli C, Franco A et al (2001) Activation of coagulation and fibrinolysis during coronary surgery: on-pump versus off-pump techniques. Anesthesiology 95:1103–1109
12. Cavarocchi NC, England MD, Schaff HV et al (1986) Oxygen free radical generation during cardiopulmonary bypass: correlation with complement activation. Circulation 74:III130–III133
13. Chenoweth DE, Cooper SW, Hugli TE, Stewart RW, Blackstone EH, Kirklin JW (1981) Complement activation during cardiopulmonary bypass: evidence for generation of C3a and C5a anaphylatoxins. N Engl J Med 304:497–503
14. de Waal M, Abrams J, Bennett B, Figdor CG, de Vries JE (1991) Interleukin 10(IL-10) inhibits cytokine synthesis by human monocytes: an autoregulatory role of IL-10 produced by monocytes. J Exp Med 174:1209–1220
15. Dehoux MS, Hernot S, Asehnoune K et al (2000) Cardiopulmonary bypass decreases cytokine production in lipopolysaccharide-stimulated whole blood cells: roles of interleukin-10 and the extracorporeal circuit. Crit Care Med 28:1721–1727
16. Diegeler A, Doll N, Rauch T et al (2000) Humoral immune response during coronary artery bypass grafting: a comparison of limited approach, "off-pump" technique, and conventional cardiopulmonary bypass. Circulation 102:III95–100
17. Diegeler A, Tarnok A, Rauch T et al (1998) Changes of leukocyte subsets in coronary artery bypass surgery: cardiopulmonary bypass versus 'off-pump' techniques. Thorac Cardiovasc Surg 46: 327–332
18. Dreyer WJ, Michael LH, Millman EE, Berens KL (1995) Neutrophil activation and adhesion molecule expression in a canine model of open heart surgery with cardiopulmonary bypass. Cardiovasc Res 29:775–781
19. Edmunds LHJ (1993) Blood-surface interactions during cardiopulmonary bypass. J Card Surg 8:404–410
20. Flohe S, Börgermann J, Dominguez FE et al (1999) Influence of granulocyte-macrophage colony-stimulating factor (GM-CSF) on whole blood endotoxin responsiveness following trauma, cardiopulmonary bypass, and severe sepsis. Shock 12:17–24

21. Fransen E, Maessen J, Dentener M, Senden N, Geskes G, Buurman W (1998) Systemic inflammation present in patients undergoing CABG without extracorporeal circulation. Chest 113:1290–1295

22. Gill M, Dias S, Hattori K et al (2001) Vascular trauma induces rapid but transient mobilization of VEGFR2(+)AC133(+) endothelial precursor cells. Circ Res 88:167–174

23. Gillinov AM, Bator JM, Zehr KJ et al (1993) Neutrophil adhesion molecule expression during cardiopulmonary bypass with bubble and membrane oxygenators. Ann Thorac Surg 56:847–853

24. Gillinov AM, Redmond JM, Winkelstein JA et al (1994) Complement and neutrophil activation during cardiopulmonary bypass: a study in the complement-deficient dog. Ann Thorac Surg 57:345–352

25. Gillinov AM, Redmond JM, Zehr KJ et al (1994) Inhibition of neutrophil adhesion during cardiopulmonary bypass. Ann Thorac Surg 57:126–133

26. Gu YJ, Mariani MA, Boonstra PW, Grandjean JG, van Oeveren W (1999) Complement activation in coronary artery bypass grafting patients without cardiopulmonary bypass: the role of tissue injury by surgical incision. Chest 116:892–898

27. Gulielmos V, Menschikowski M, Dill H et al (2000) Interleukin-1, interleukin-6 and myocardial enzyme response after coronary artery bypass grafting – a prospective randomized comparison of the conventional and three minimally invasive surgical techniques. Eur J Cardiothorac Surg 18:594–601

28. Hall RI, Smith MS, Rocker G (1997) The systemic inflammatory response to cardiopulmonary bypass: pathophysiological, therapeutic, and pharmacological considerations. Anesth Analg 85:766–782

29. Ilton MK, Langton PE, Taylor ML et al (1999) Differential expression of neutrophil adhesion molecules during coronary artery surgery with cardiopulmonary bypass. J Thorac Cardiovasc Surg 118:930–937

30. Kawamura T, Wakusawa R, Okada K, Inada S (1993) Elevation of cytokines during open heart surgery with cardiopulmonary bypass: participation of interleukin 8 and 6 in reperfusion injury. Can J Anaesth 40:1016–1021

31. Kirklin JK, Westaby S, Blackstone EH, Kirklin JW, Chenoweth DE, Pacifico AD (1983) Complement and the damaging effects of cardiopulmonary bypass. J Thorac Cardiovasc Surg 86:845–857

32. Kukielka GL, Smith CW, LaRosa GJ et al (1995) Interleukin-8 gene induction in the myocardium after ischemia and reperfusion in vivo. J Clin Invest 95:89–103

33. Mangano DT (2002) Aspirin and mortality from coronary bypass surgery. N Engl J Med 347:1309–1317

34. Mariani MA, Gu YJ, Boonstra PW, Grandjean JG, van Oeveren W, Ebels T (1999) Procoagulant activity after off-pump coronary operation: is the current anticoagulation adequate? Ann Thorac Surg 67:1370–1375

35. Markewitz A, Faist E, Lang S, Endres S, Hultner L, Reichart B (1993) Regulation of acute phase response after cardiopulmonary bypass by immunomodulation. Ann Thorac Surg 55:389–394

36. Matata BM, Sosnowski AW, Galinanes M (2000) Off-pump bypass graft operation significantly reduces oxidative stress and inflammation. Ann Thorac Surg 69:785–791

37. Menasche P, Peynet J, Lariviere J et al (1994)Does normothermia during cardiopulmonary bypass increase neutrophil-endothelium interactions? Circulation 90:II275–279

38. Moore FDJ, Warner KG, Assousa S, Valeri CR, Khuri SF (1988) The effects of complement activation during cardiopulmonary bypass. Attenuation by hypothermia, heparin, and hemodilution. Ann Surg 208:95–103

39. Naldini A, Borrelli E, Cesari S, Giomarelli P, Toscano M (1995) In vitro cytokine production and T-cell proliferation in patients undergoing cardiopulmonary by-pass. Cytokine 7:165–170

40. Neufeld G, Cohen T, Gengrinovitch S, Poltorak Z (1999) Vascular endothelial growth factor (VEGF) and its receptors. FASEB J 13:9–22

41. Nguyen DM, Mulder DS, Shennib H (1992) Effect of cardiopulmonary bypass on circulating lymphocyte function. Ann Thorac Surg 53:611–616

42. Randow F, Syrbe U, Meisel C et al (1995) Mechanism of endotoxin desensitization: involvement of interleukin 10 and transforming growth factor beta. J Exp Med 181:1887–1892

43. Rinder CS, Bonan JL, Rinder HM, Mathew J, Hines R, Smith BR (1992) Cardiopulmonary bypass induces leukocyte-platelet adhesion. Blood 79:1201–1205

44. Schulze C, Conrad N, Schutz A et al (2000) Reduced expression of systemic proinflammatory cytokines after off-pump versus conven-

tional coronary artery bypass grafting. Thorac Cardiovasc Surg 48:364–369

45. Seghaye MC, Duchateau J, Bruniaux J et al (1996) Interleukin-10 release related to cardiopulmonary bypass in infants undergoing cardiac operations. J Thorac Cardiovasc Surg 111:545–553

46. Seghaye MC, Duchateau J, Grabitz RG et al (1993) Complement activation during cardiopulmonary bypass in infants and children. Relation to postoperative multiple system organ failure. J Thorac Cardiovasc Surg 106:978–987

47. Struber M, Cremer JT, Gohrbandt B et al (1999) Human cytokine responses to coronary artery bypass grafting with and without cardiopulmonary bypass. Ann Thorac Surg 68:1330–1335

48. van Dijk D, Nierich AP, Jansen EW et al (2001) Early outcome after off-pump versus on-pump coronary bypass surgery: results from a randomized study. Circulation 104:1761–1766

49. Wan S, DeSmet JM, Barvais L, Goldstein M, Vincent JL, LeClerc JL (1996) Myocardium is a major source of proinflammatory cytokines in patients undergoing cardiopulmonary bypass. J Thorac Cardiovasc Surg 112:806–811

50. Wan S, Izzat MB, Lee TW, Wan IY, Tang NL, Yim AP (1999) Avoiding cardiopulmonary bypass in multivessel CABG reduces cytokine response and myocardial injury. Ann Thorac Surg 68:52–56

51. Wan S, LeClerc JL, Schmartz D et al (1997) Hepatic release of interleukin-10 during cardiopulmonary bypass in steroid-pretreated patients. Am Heart J 133:335–339

52. Wan S, LeClerc JL, Vincent JL (1997) Cytokine responses to cardiopulmonary bypass: lessons learned from cardiac transplantation. Ann Thorac Surg 63:269–276

53. Wan S, LeClerc JL, Vincent JL (1997) Inflammatory response to cardiopulmonary bypass: mechanisms involved and possible therapeutic strategies. Chest 112:676–692

54. Wildhirt SM, Schulze C, Conrad N et al (2000) Reduced myocardial cellular damage and lipid peroxidation in off-pump versus conventional coronary artery bypass grafting. Eur J Med Res 5:222–228

55. Wildhirt SM, Schulze C, Schulz C et al (2001) Reduction of systemic and cardiac adhesion molecule expression after off-pump versus conventional coronary artery bypass grafting. Shock 16 Suppl 1:55–59

56. Yang Z, Zingarelli B, Szabo C (2000) Crucial role of endogenous interleukin-10 production in myocardial ischemia/reperfusion injury. Circulation 101:1019–1026
57. Youker KA, Hawkins HK, Kukielka GL et al (1994) Molecular evidence for induction of intracellular adhesion molecule-1 in the viable border zone associated with ischemia-reperfusion injury of the dog heart. Circulation 89:2736–2746

CHAPTER 2 OPCAB

Different stabilizer concepts and exposure techniques for off-pump coronary artery bypass surgery

C. Detter, T. Deuse

Introduction

Coronary artery revascularization on the beating heart without the use of cardiopulmonary bypass (CPB) involves a more technically challenging anastomosis. Stabilizers are a major tool in OPCAB procedures, reducing the cardiac surface motion during suturing of the anastomosis. Initial attempts with multiple stay sutures, vessel loops, slings, and pharmacological movement adaptation with adenosine or other pharmacological agents [10] were successful but left a significant number of anastomotic stenoses or bypass occlusions (10%). The major limitation of these techniques was the residual cardiac surface motion, which may hamper the meticulous construction of the distal anastomosis. Thus, different cardiac surface stabilizers were developed for local cardiac immobilization, which improved early angiographic results markedly [8]. To reduce cardiac movement sufficiently, three different stabilizer concepts are available: 1) pressure stabilizers, 2) suction stabilizers, and 3) the platform technique (Fig. 1). Despite growing enthusiasm, these techniques were used almost exclusively in patients with coronary artery disease limited to the left anterior descending (LAD) artery. Revascularization of other coronary territories remained elusive because of technical difficulties with hemodynamic instability in exposing the lateral and inferior wall of the heart.

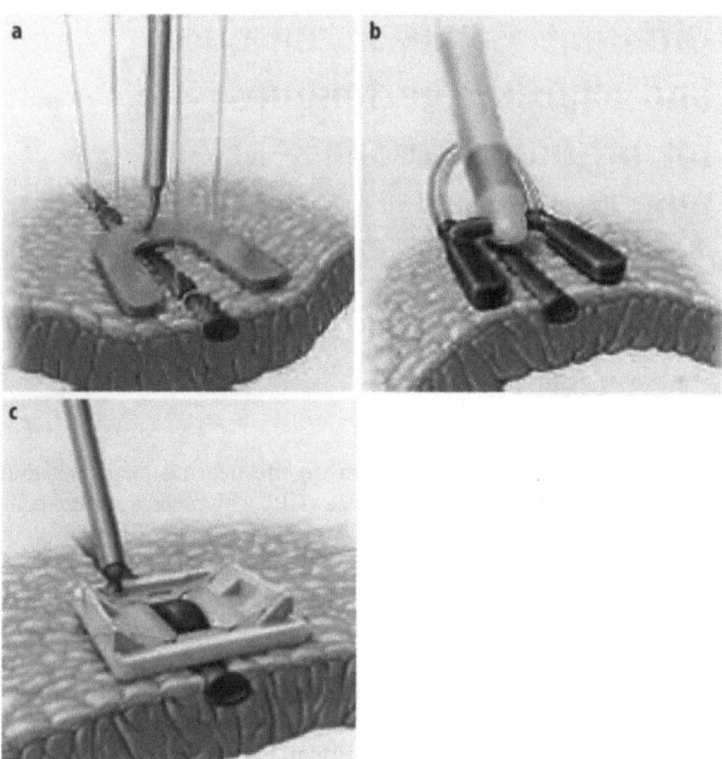

Fig. 1. A drawing of the three different stabilizer concepts comparing pressure stabilizers (**a**), suction stabilizers (**b**), and the platform technique (**c**)

This chapter describes strategies and techniques of coronary exposure and different stabilizer concepts. In particular, advantages, disadvantages, and possible pitfalls are discussed in detail.

Stabilizer concepts

The pressure stabilizing concept

A U-shaped metal blade is pressed onto the cardiac surface to achieve epicardial stabilization. A rigid arm, fixed at the sternum retractor, positions the blade. The stabilizer is adjusted and locked in place, centering the coronary vessel between the tines of the "horse-shoe" of the stabilizer. The pressure is carefully adjusted not to compromise ventricular function.

This concept is widely used for stabilization of the left anterior descending artery in MIDCAB surgery [1]. Major advantages are the simple concept and the minimal space required, an advantage in limited incisions. However, they do cause pressure on the ventricle which may adversely affect ventricular function and they have only very limited rotation/presentation function [11].

The suction stabilizing concept

Local stabilization can be achieved by suction onto the heart surface. There are different stabilizers commercially available:

The Axius™ device

The Axius™ Vacuum Stabilizer System (Guidant Corporation, Santa Clara, CA) is a new family of vacuum stabilization devices. Choices in vacuum stabilization include the Axius Vacuum Stabilizer with Rigid (–275 mmHg) or the Axius Vacuum Stabilizer with Malleable Feet (–400 mmHg) for optimal stabilization, enhanced anastomotic site access with improved visibility, and greater ease of use. Both Guidant Axius Vacuum Stabilizer Systems consist of the AccessRail™ Platform and the Axius™ Vacuum Stabilizer. The AccessRail Platform is attached onto a reusable Activator™ Drive Mechanism. The AccessRail Platform, along with an Activator Drive Mechanism, is designed to create surgical access to, and direct visualization of, the thoracic cavity through a sternotomy incision. The AccessRail Platform also allows for the organization of the pericardial sutures. The AccessRail Platform accommodates the Axius Vacuum Stabilizer with Rigid or the Axius™ Vacuum Stabilizer with Malleable Feet, which consists of a Flexi-Link™ low profile arm with an articulating foot at the distal end and a mount that connects to the AccessRail Platform. The stabilizer provides local immobilization of the target vessel on the beating heart. This system is designed to perform total off-pump coronary revascularization.

The Octopus® device

The first commercially available suction stabilizer was the Octopus 1 tissue stabilizer system (Medtronic Inc., Minneapolis, MN), which consists of two suction paddles with four or five suction domes on each paddle [2]. Each paddle-handle was connected with a rigid holding arm to the operating table rail. A simple straight paddle was used in the lengthwise approach to the vessel. Left and right versions allowed placement of the low-profile side facing the coronary artery to provide optimal access for construction of the anastomosis.

Meanwhile, the Octopus 4 tissue stabilizer is available. This new device is much smaller and allows more flexible handling. It can be fixed to any site of the rail on the sternum retractor. The low profile arm stays out of surgeon's field of vision and its flexibility allows customized placement. The two feet carrying the suction domes are no longer rigid, but malleable for maximum engagement with the epicardial surface.

One major advantage of the suction stabilizing concept is the ability of easy readjustment at the anastomotic site by switching off the suction and repositioning the device. Thus, the vessel can easily be dissected over a longer distance for detection of the optimal target area for coronary anastomosis. The suction devices have a dual role, first to immobilize the heart by lifting and thereby reducing pressure on the ventricle, and second to rotate or present the heart.

▌ The platform stabilizing concept

The Immobilizer™ system (Genzyme Surgical Products, Cambridge, MA) uses a flexible arm, comparable to those mentioned above, to position the platform at the anastomotic site. Epicardial stabilization is then achieved by capturing the target vessel with gentle epicardial herniation through the anastomotic window of the Cohn platform. Vessel loops are utilized to provide atraumatic, anterior-posterior compression and to achieve hemostasis. The loops are placed underneath the coronary vessels and are fixed to the platform. Thus, besides stabilization, a clear and bloodless field is achieved. Additional sutures surrounding the coronary arteries proximally to the region of the anastomosis to achieve temporary interruption of blood flow are not necessary. Be sure not to press the platform onto the cardiac surface. This is not necessary and may cause hemodynamic compromization.

With this device, the two-dimensional cardiac surface motion can most efficiently be reduced [4]. A disadvantage of this concept may be that movements of the platform along the target vessel require repositioning of the vessel loops. After fixation of the vessel loops, the Immobilizer™ is less flexible and readjustment is inconvenient. To facilitate dissection of the coronary vessel, the distal part of the platform should be removed and the device should be used as a U-shaped "pressure" stabilizer. If the target area is found, a new platform is used and the vessel loops are placed to perform the anastomosis.

Exposure of the heart

For total myocardial revascularization without CPB on the beating heart, a full sternotomy is the incision of choice. In the early era of OPCAB surgery, revascularization of all territories of the heart was difficult because of the needed luxation of the heart. To expose the lateral and inferior wall of the heart, different techniques are available:

▌ Pericardial sutures

The heart can be exposed by placing multiple sutures in the posterior pericardium. The pericardial sutures are placed between the left upper and lower pulmonary veins and at the diaphragm. These are referred to as Lima sutures after Ricardo Lima from Brazil. By pulling these sutures, the heart can be elevated and rotated.

▌ The "single suture" technique

The "single suture" technique represents a modification of exposing the heart by placing pericardial sutures. This technique involves elevation of the beating heart and placement of a heavy suture (No. 1, Ethibond, Ethicon Inc, Somerville, NJ) in the oblique sinus of the posterior pericardium between the right and left inferior pulmonary veins. The suture is then passed through a folded vaginal tape and snared down to the posterior pericardium using a tourniquet [9]. Exposure of various coronary territories is obtained by using different combinations of elevation and lateral displacement. This can be accomplished by adjusting the orientation of both vaginal tape and snares, and by applying various degree of traction. Be sure to avoid circumferential compression. This would impair cardiac function by alteration of the geometry of the cardiac chambers.

▌ Heart positioners

To achieve sufficient heart luxation with minimal ventricular deterioration, heart positioners were developed. Meanwhile, different devices are offered in combination with suction- or platform stabilizers to achieve both, myocardial stabilization and heart positioning.

Xpose™ Access Device

The Axius™ off-pump system (Guidant Corporation) was the first complete system on the market to offer stabilization and access technologies (Fig. 2). In the meantime the fourth generation is available. The Xpose™ Access Device is designed to securely lift the heart during off-pump bypass surgery and easily position and access target vessels, while maintaining hemodynamics. Designed for both apical and non-apical placement on the heart, this access device features a low profile link arm for exceptional maneuverability, greater access and ease of use. The arm is attached to the AccessRail™ Platform with the Quick-Lock Knob and can be placed at any point of the retractor to allow positioning of the heart. After the cup is positioned apical or non-apical on the heart, suction is applied through the

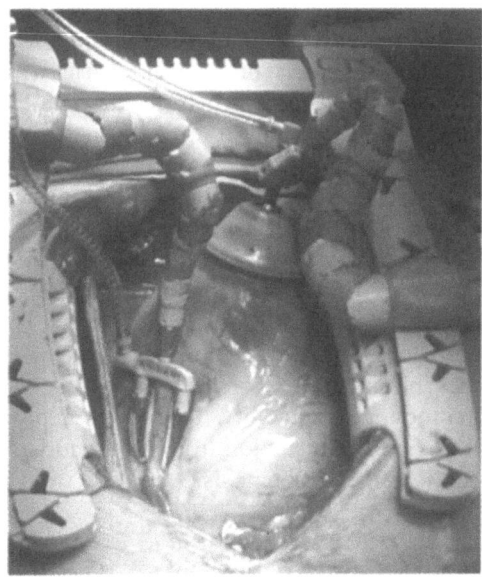

Fig. 2. The Axius™ off-pump system with Axius™ Vacuum 2 Stabilizer and Xpose™ 3 Access Device

cup to allow capturing of the heart with normal cardiac motion. The vacuum source is regulated to a vacuum pressure of –250 mmHg.

The Starfish™ Heart Positioner

The Starfish™ Heart Positioner (Medtronic Inc.) consists of an articulating arm with a multi-appendage, silicone suction cup attached to a flexible headlink system minimizing restriction of cardiac motion (Fig. 3). The arm is fixed at the stabilizer retractor and can also be placed at any point on the retractor. Instead of applying the device to the apex as with the Xpose device, the Starfish™ can also be attached lateral to the apex to enhance lateral wall exposure.

The Immobilizer™ Heart Manipulation Device

The Immobilizer™ Heart Manipulation Device (Genzyme Corporation) consists of a flexible arm with a malleable suction cup similar to the Starfish device. The Heart Manipulation Device is attached to the apex or the posterior-lateral wall position.

These devices allow heart positioning to facilitate access to all vessels without compromising diastolic ventricular relaxation as seen with manual luxation techniques. After placing the cup to or next to the apex and starting suction, the luxation is slowly adjusted and the arm is locked. The flexibility of the cup and its ability to easily rotate at the wrist of the arm guarantees minimal deterioration of cardiac function and preserves hemodynamic stability. Be sure to reposition the heart before turning off the suction to avoid a sudden drop of the heart that can tear the anastomosis.

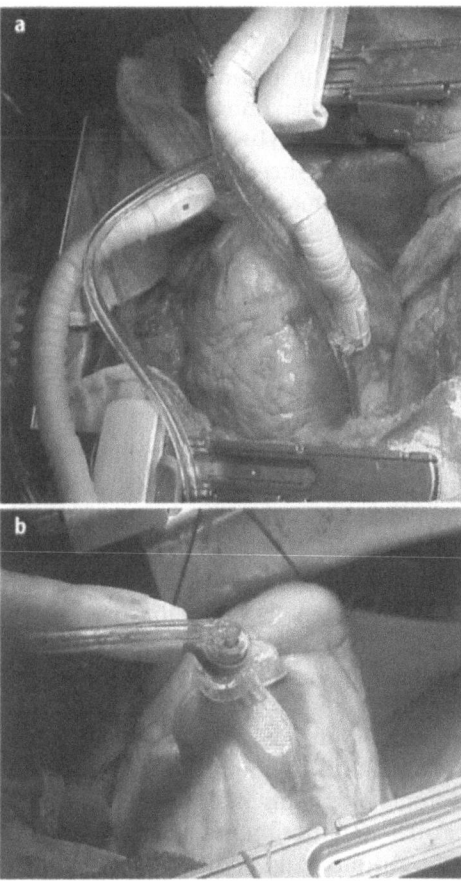

Fig. 3. The Octopus® System with Octopus® Tissue Stabilizer (**a**) and Starfish Heart Positioner (**b**)

Summary

Stabilizers have shown to be useful in off-pump surgery, reducing the cardiac surface motion during suturing of the anastomosis. Borst et al. could demonstrate a wall motion reduction to 1×1 mm with the Octopus® 1 stabilizer [2]. The new generation of stabilizers is even more effective as shown in a recent study [4]. The two-dimensional cardiac surface motion is reduced to a maximum deviation of 423.5 ± 129.6 µm with the Octopus 3 and 109.7 ± 32.4 µm with the Immobilizer device. Furthermore, these stabilizing devices were likely to result in a substantial improvement of angiographic results. Possati et al. could show that patients operated using a stabilizer device had angiographic results clearly superior to those of patients operated without stabilization with a perfect patency rate of 100% versus 81.8% [8]. Calafiore and colleagues report results of 261 patients before and after the stabilization era [3]. Early angiography in patients who were studied before the utilization of stabilization devices revealed a patency rate of 92.5% versus 98.8% with the use of a stabilizer ($p = 0.026$), the perfect patency rate was 90.3% versus 97.6%, respectively ($p = 0.031$). Subramanian and associates report on improvement in the patency rate from 89% to 97% ($p = 0.055$) after the routine use of mechanical stabilizing devices [12].

The development of stabilizers was a crucial step in the beginning of off-pump surgery. Now a variety of stabilizers are available in an attempt to improve exposure and stabilization of coronary targets in OPCAB surgery. These stabilizers represent different strategies of cardiac stabilization and vessel occlusion. Due to technical improvements, access to all vessels is possible. Complete systems offering both heart manipulation and myocardial stabilization are available. With heart positioners, cardiac positioning is additionally simplified, which facilitates the access and exposure of coronary arteries [5, 7]. This minimizes the associated hemodynamic deterioration especially when compared to deep pericardial sutures for lateral and posterior wall revascularization [6]. Thus, total revascularization on the beating heart has become possible and OPCAB surgery can be offered to a wide patient population.

References

1. Boonstra PW, Grandjean JG, Mariani MA (1997) Improved method for direct coronary grafting without CPB via anterolateral small thoracotomy. Ann Thorac Surg 63:567–569
2. Borst C, Jansen EW, Tulleken CA, Gründeman PF, Beck HJ (1996) Coronary artery bypass grafting without cardiopulmonary bypass and without interruption of native coronary flow using a novel anastomosis site restraining device ("Octopus"). J Am Coll Cardiol 27:1356–1364
3. Calafiore AM, Vitolla G, Mazzei V, Teodori G, Di Giammarco G, Iovino T, Iaco A (1998) The LAST operation: techniques and results before and after the stabilization era. Ann Thorac Surg 66:998–1001
4. Detter C, Deuse T, Christ F, Boehm DH, Reichenspurner H, Reichart B (2002) Comparison of two stabilizer concepts for off-pump coronary artery bypass grafting. Ann Thorac Surg 74:497–501
5. Dullum MK, Resano FG (2000) Xpose: a new device that provides reproducible and easy access for multivessel beating heart bypass grafting. Heart Surg Forum 3:113–118
6. Grundeman P, et al (2002) Ninety degrees anterior cardiac displacement in off-pump CABG: the Starfish™ cardiac positioner preserves stroke volume and anterior pressure. Presented at ISMICS
7. Niinami H, Takeuchi Y, Ichikawa S, Ban T, Higashita R, Suda Y, Yamamoto M (2002) Multivessel off-pump coronary aortic bypass grafting with an impaired and severely dilated left ventricle using the Starfish heart positioner. Kyobu Geka 55:773–777
8. Possati G, Gaudino M, Alessandrini F, Zimarino M, Glieca F, Luciani N (1998) Systematic clinical and angiographic follow-up of patients undergoing minimally invasive coronary artery bypass. J Thorac Cardiovasc Surg 115:785–790
9. Ricci M, Karamanoukian HL, D'Ancona G, Bergsland J, Salerno TA (2000) Exposure and mechanical stabilization in off-pump coronary artery bypass grafting via sternotomy. Ann Thorac Surg 70:1736–1740
10. Robinson MC, Thielmeier KA, Hill BB (1997) Transient ventricular asystole using adenosine during minimally invasive and open sternotomy coronary artery bypass grafting. Ann Thorac Surg 63 (6 Suppl):S30–34
11. Stanbridge RD, Hadjinikolaou LK (1999) Technical adjuncts in beating heart surgery comparison of MIDCAB to off-pump sternotomy: a meta-analysis. Eur J Cardiothorac Surg16(Suppl 2):S24–33
12. Subramanian VA, McCabe JC, Geller CM (1997) Minimally invasive direct coronary artery bypass grafting: two-year clinical experience. Ann Thorac Surg 64:1648–1655

Adjunct tools in OPCAB surgery

I. Friedrich, J. Börgermann

Introduction

No matter what the specific technique, constructing perfect anastomoses remains the basic prerequisite for successful coronary revascularization. During an OPCAB procedure, the following steps are required to construct an adequate anastomosis: 1) ensure stable cardiovascular dynamics, 2) obtain ergonomically favorable exposure of the target area, 3) guarantee optimal stabilization of the cardiac surface without compromising hemodynamic stability, 4) expose the coronary vessel in a practically bloodless manner while avoiding any ischemic response. Beating-heart procedures are much more challenging for the surgeon than operations on the arrested heart. By now an extensive arsenal of surgical tools has become available to support surgeons in their technically demanding endeavor. Topics such as techniques for intraoperative stabilization of the heart and the benefit of using a pacemaker with epicardial electrodes are comprehensively covered in other chapters.

IABP

Patients with severely reduced ventricular function or an acute myocardial infarction will often require insertion of an intraaortic balloon catheter as a prerequisite for undergoing surgery using the OPCAB method [1]. Numerous publications support the favorable hemodynamic effects of IABP. Decreased afterload and increased diastolic blood pressure improve myocardial perfusion, with a subsequent reduction of wall tension and increased cardiac output, on the one hand, and therefore lowered filling pressures, on the other. Even if randomized studies on IABP use for OPCAB procedures are still pending, one should consider IABP insertion in high-risk patients.

Intracoronary shunts

The use of intracoronary shunts can have a crucial impact on maintaining hemodynamic stability. Shunts help avoid ischemic reactions and hemodynamic deterioration that might necessitate conversion, especially when dealing with large caliber coronary arteries which provide retrograde flow to occluded not-bypassable areas (Fig. 1). Hemodynamic parameters such as

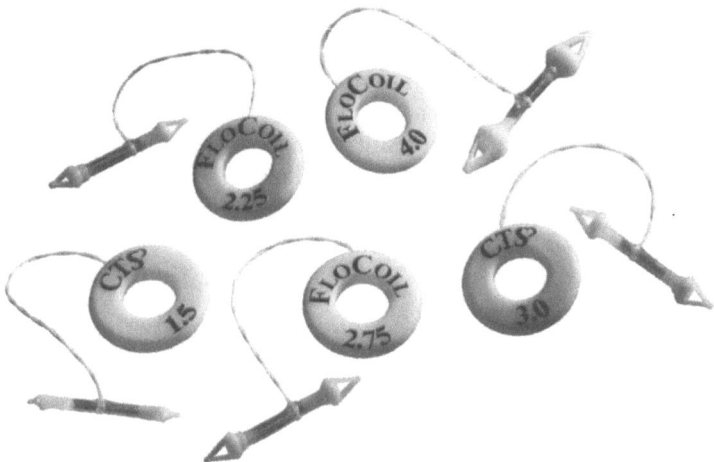

Fig. 1. Intracoronary shunts

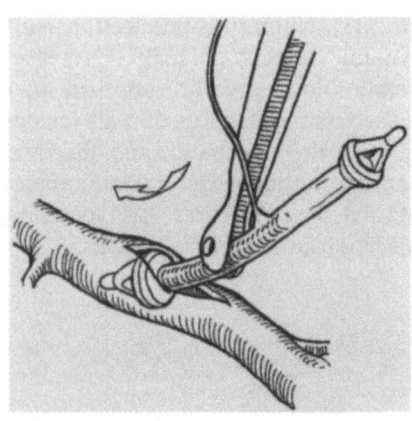

Fig. 2. Insertion of IC-shunts

stroke volume, filling pressures, and cardiac index are much more affected when the coronary arteries are simply snared as opposed to when intracoronary shunts are inserted. Shunts help to provide quick hemodynamic recovery after the distal anastomoses are completed, particular in the circumflex area, whereas hemodynamics tend to remain compromised after sole snaring of the coronary artery [5]. We do not intend to withhold that constructing the anastomosis is technically more difficult with a shunt in place than without a shunt (Figs. 2 and 3). In addition, dissection of the coronary artery or detachment of an atheromatous plaque as a result of shunt placement are serious issues. Overall, the advantages of shunt placement appear to predominate.

Snares

Occluding a severely calcified vessel is tricky. Snaring can often be avoided if an intracoronary shunt is placed. If a shunt does not control bleeding from the incised coronary artery, it is advisable to place a proximal vessel loop. For this, only soft silas-

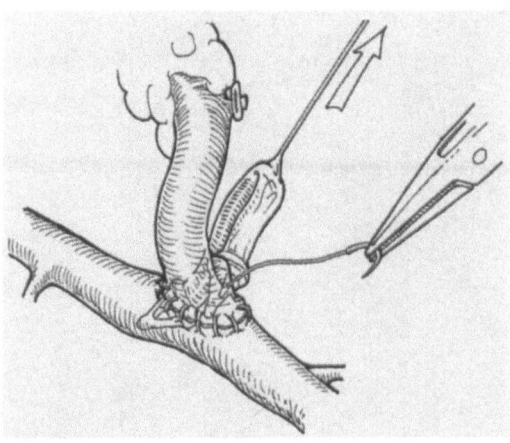

Fig. 3. Removal of IC-shunts

tic tubes should be used to minimize coronary artery trauma. Distal snaring, which could lead to endothelial damage and subsequent stenosis distal to the anastomosis, should be avoided as a matter of principle.

Blower/mister

A blower/mister delivers a spray of saline/CO_2 into the incised coronary vessel to provide clear visualization of the coronary artery (Fig. 4). When distal snaring of the vessel is avoided, considerable retrograde bleeding can impair visualization of the coronary lumen. Technically adequate grafting of the LAD may also be impeded by marked bleeding from septal branches. One needs to note that high mister flow rates and bringing the mister too close to the vessel may lead to dissection of the coronary artery. An additional critical comment concerns the fact that the long-term effects of high carbon dioxide concentrations on the coronary endothelium remain to be investigated.

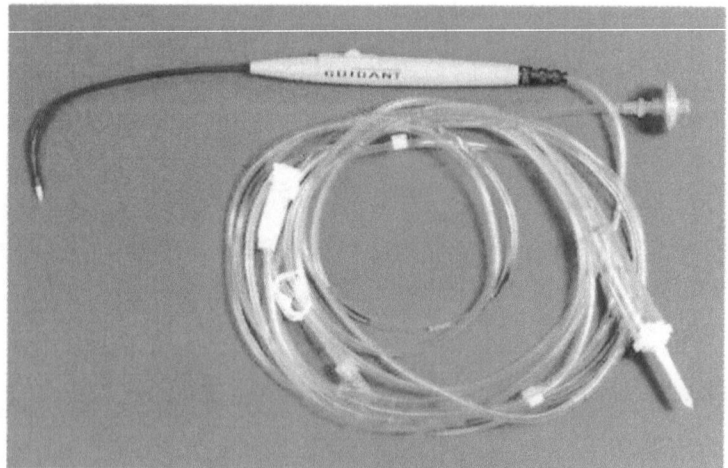

Fig. 4. Blower/mister

When air is used instead of CO_2, there is a risk that significant amounts of air embolized into the coronary artery.

Epiaortic sonography

Clamping the ascending aorta can detach intracoronary atheromatous plaques. The use of epiaortic sonography permits localization of such plaques so that the proximal anastomoses can be performed in different areas, distant from intravascular pathology.

Proximal anastomotic devices

For high-risk patients with a severely calcified ascending aorta, proximal anastomotic devices are now available (Fig. 5). They

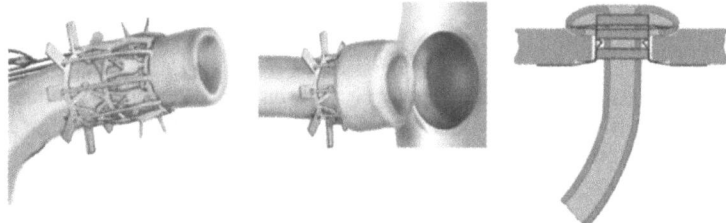

Fig. 5. Proximal anastomotic devices, Guidant Inc

are useful if T and composite grafts are not feasible [3]. If the use of these devices does in fact reduce the risk of stroke has not be demonstrated so far. In additional, no quantitative data are available yet regarding the risk of complications from these devices.

Flow meter

Due to the more challenging technical requirements of beating-heart revascularization, one should assess all results from a self-critical perspective and demand objective quality control. This includes the intraoperative evaluation of graft patency and – should problems arise in the intensive care unit – liberal indications for postoperative coronary angiography. Various methods for evaluating graft flow are currently in clinical use; the transit time method is the most widely used technique. The interpretation of measurement results is strongly dependent on the user's experience, however. VANHIMBERGEN et al. review the technique and its limitations and provide an in-depth discussion of the often difficult issue of distinguishing a stenosis at the distal anastomosis vs. other factors such as competitive flow or diffuse distal coronary stenoses [2, 4]. Despite all limitations, it appears that one should not do without intraoperative flow measurements to ensure the utmost quality of surgical care.

References

1. Craver JM, Murrah CP (2001) Elective intraaortic balloon counter-pulsation for high-risk off-pump coronary artery bypass operations. Ann Thorac Surg 71(4):1220–1223
2. D'Ancona G, Karamanoukian HL, Ricci M, Schmid S, Bergsland J, Salerno TA (2000) Graft revision after transit time flow measurement in off-pump coronary artery bypass grafting. Eur J Cardio-thorac Surg 7(3):287–293
3. Eckstein FS, Bonilla LF, Englberger L, Stauffer E, Berg TA, Schmidli J et al (2001) Minimizing aortic manipulation during OPCAB using the symmetry aortic connector system for proximal vein graft ana-stomoses. Ann Thorac Surg 72(3):S995–S998
4. Van Himbergen DJ, Koenig SC, Jaber SF, Cerrito PB, Spence PA (1999) A review of transit-time flow measurement for assessing graft patency. Heart Surg Forum 2(3):226–229
5. Yeatman M, Caputo M, Narayan P, Ghosh AK, Ascione R, Ryder I et al (2002) Intracoronary shunts reduce transient intraoperative myo-cardial dysfunction during off-pump coronary operations. Ann Thorac Surg 73(5):1411–1417

Monitoring and devices for hemodynamic assessment during OPCAB

A. P. Nierich, J. Damen

Introduction

Monitoring is aimed to cope with the disturbances of the physiology of the patient during surgery and anesthesia in order to prevent harm to the patient. Patient monitoring is a key aspect of anesthesiology, and anesthesiologists should be able to interpret and evaluate the clinical relevance of changes and to react properly to a change in physiologic parameters. It is the challenging task of the anesthesiologist, as the primary perioperative care provider to identify patients with unstable or high-risk conditions and insure adequate care prior, during and following surgery. OPCAB surgery is basically different from other surgery. One can consider OPCAB as 'repairing the engine of a car while driving on the highway'. Everyone feels that this might be not so easy and could lead to problems for the engine, car and/or mechanic. The same is true for OPCAB: clamping native coronary arteries might induce ischemia or cardiac fibrillation; cardiac dislocation might lead to an impaired systemic circulation; inadequate motion reduction of the epicardium might result in problems with the vascular anastomosis.

Cardiac repositioning is necessary in order to reach all sides of the heart during OPCAB. This results in changes in the coronary circulation. Several animal and human studies have demonstrated impaired biventricular function, especially right

Table 1. Review of studies focused on hemodynamic changes during OPCAB related to positioning of the heart

Variable	LAD positioning			Trend LAD	PDA positioning			Trend PDA	Cx positioning			Trend Cx
	Nierich [24] N=96	Watters [34] N=29	Mathison [19] N=42		Nierich [24] N=84	Watters [34] N=15	Mathison [19] N=24		Nierich [24] N=37	Watters [34] N=21	Mathison [19] N=44	
HR	9	3	8	+	10	4	6	+	11	4	16	+
MAP	-4	-3	-4	=	-7	-6	-10	-	-6	-5	-18	-
RAP	10	8	9	+	0	42	52	++	-6	-5	-18	-
mPAP	6	9	nv	+	-6	14	nv	=	10	53	89	++
PCWP	nv	41	16	++	nv	27	24	++	nv	37	45	++
CO	-4	-9	-18	-	-4	-20	-21	-	-8	-25	-36	-
SV	-4	-16	-17	-	-17	-24	-34	-	-18	-28	-48	-
SvO_2	-3	nv	-8	=	0	nv	-13	-	-6	nv	-16	-

Values are % change compared to baseline before manipulation of the heart.
LAD left anterior descending; PDA posterior descending artery; Cx circumflex artery; HR heart rate; MAP mean arterial pressure; RAP right atrial pressure; mPAP mean pulmonary artery pressure; PCWP pulmonary capillary wedge pressure; CO cardiac output; SV Stroke volume; SvO_2 mixed venous oxygen saturation; nv no value or not performed
Trend abbreviations: =: change between -5% and +5%; +: change between +5% and +20%; ++: change > +20%;
-: change between -5% and -20%; -: change >-20%

ventricular dysfunction, during cardiac displacement [12, 14, 18, 24]. This appears to be secondary to deformation of the cardiac chambers. During lateral and vertical displacement, the heart appears to buckle, resulting in compression of the right ventricle between the pericardium and the interventricular septum, which in turn reduces left ventricular filling and cardiac output. Table 1 summarizes the clinical human studies [19, 24, 34] that focused especially on hemodynamic changes during OPCAB on the three main sites of the heart: anterior, lateral and inferior wall. These clinical situations make adequate anesthetic management and monitoring essential for good surgical performance [25].

The communication between surgeon and anesthesiologist is the key to the success of OPCAB surgery. A proactive anesthesiologist in this type of surgery will allow the surgeon to concentrate on the difficult revascularization task. There should be a constant feedback of hemodynamic changes during the different surgical phases. The anesthesiologist should keep the surgeon informed about the use of inotropes or vasopressors, ST segment or rhythm disturbances, and the patient's general condition. Also, the surgeon should communicate with the anesthesiologist when the heart is being displaced, when a coronary artery is occluded, and whether a shunt is used or not. In no other cardiac procedure is it more important for the anesthesiologist to continually observe and treat the hemodynamic and rhythm responses to cardiac manipulation and regional ischemia.

Monitoring in OPCAB

Hemodynamics

The American Society of Anesthesiology suggests that standard monitors and arterial lines are needed during beating heart surgery. Central vascular access is also necessary for the administration of vasoactive drugs and monitoring. Additional monitoring depends not only on the comorbidity of the patient but also on the extent of the surgical procedure. During the beginning of OPCAB surgery, extensive monitoring was used in order to study and learn what the impact of OPCAB would be, not only on the heart but especially on other organ systems [25]. Nowadays, after the learning phase, monitoring is tailored for each case but is still extensive in case of research. Types of additional monitoring include the use of a pulmonary artery catheter (PAC), non-invasive cardiac output methods, transesophageal echocardiography (TEE) and transcranial Doppler (TCD).

∎ ECG, particularly ST segment changes.

For ischemic monitoring, the electrocardiogram (ECG) is critical but also has important limitations if the heart is tilted. The use of pericardial slings, cardiac stabilization and positioning devices all lead to displacement of the heart. This alters the appearance of the ECG, which often decreases in amplitude and axis. In this situation, the ST segment changes may be falsely minimized, when in fact they represent 50% of the ECG complex. Usually, ECG monitoring during posterior wall revascularization is of little value [24, 32]. Research in the recent years has focused on the early and accurate detection of myocardial ischemia in order to start treatment as early as possible. There are, however, no studies showing that the early diagnosis and subsequent treatment affects the cardiac outcome of non-cardiac surgery. Despite the lack of data, perioperative myocardial ischemia should be treated aggressively until the contrary has been proven.

∎ Swan-Ganz or pulmonary artery catheter (PAC) (with CCO/SvO$_2$ monitoring).

The use of PAC has several advantages, although the debate whether or not the PAC influences outcome still goes on even after 30 years. It is a quantitative diagnostic tool of global circulation. Pressure monitoring allows optimizing pre-load to the heart elevations in PAP or PCWP are indicative for myocardial ischemia. However, the combination of measuring cardiac output by thermodilution or continuously (CCO) with mixed venous oxygen saturation (SvO_2) gives the opportunity, not only to optimize hemodynamics for the heart but also to control global circulation for the rest of the body. The addition of continuous monitoring of cardiac output instead of intermittent measurement by thermodilution has increased simplicity of the device. Accuracy of the continuous technique is comparable with the thermodilution method [4, 20, 36]. The CCO method is, however, often too slow to give a good impression of fast hemodynamic changes during OPCAB.

The addition of SvO_2 monitoring is important as a tool to measure oxygen extraction rates [7, 22]. It generally reflects the need of the peripheral tissues of oxygen, which depends on oxygen delivery and cardiac output. The advantage is that SvO_2 reacts directly during changes and it is related to CO if the levels of oxygen delivery, consumption and hemoglobin concentration remain constant during manipulation of the heart. This gives the anesthesiologist a quantitative tool to determine the limits and balance between oxygen delivery, cardiac function and tissue oxygenation. It is especially useful if global cardiac function is already compromised and dislocation of the heart is planned. Balancing between the minimum of cardiac workload and accepting a minimum of the compromised global circulation is possible. Without this tool, one might enter into dangerously low cardiac output levels without notice. This might lead to adverse organ function postoperatively. A practical safe lower limit of SvO_2 is 60%, since gut ischemia is initiated if SvO_2 falls below 50%. However, the catheter can migrate during compression of the right ventricle during tilting and may give false high levels of SvO_2. Also, there is no relationship with improved outcome with this type of monitoring [16]. The advantage of the method is, however, automatic and will not distract the anesthesiologist from the surgical procedure.

Non-invasive cardiac output methods.

There are several systems now available that are suitable to use during OPCAB, in order to measure CO. Clinical evaluation in OPCAB is ongoing.

Pulse-contour CO is computed by measuring the area under the arterial pressure waveform and dividing it by aortic impedance. Aortic impedance is determined by an arterial thermodilution at the onset of the system. Arterial pulse-contour analysis is easy to use and minimally invasive, thus, qualifies as a reliable routine monitoring tool during minimally invasive coronary surgery with tissue stabilizers [11].

Cardiac output is often monitored after cardiac operations with a PAC. A new method has been introduced that measures cardiac output by lithium dilution (LiDCO) and uses these data to calibrate a system (PulseCO) that calculates cardiac output continuously from the energy of the arterial pressure waveform [15].

A non-invasive cardiac output monitor (NICO) based on partial CO_2 rebreathing technique and a modified Fick equation is another method. Clinical evaluation shows that partial CO_2 rebreathing technique provides a useful and accurate non-invasive estimate of cardiac output. However, reaction time during acute CO changes needs further evaluation [27].

▌ Transesophageal echocardiography (TEE).

TEE is a rapidly evolving technique and requires specific interpretation skills. Practice guidelines for the use of perioperative use of TEE have been described [31]. TEE is used as a qualitative diagnostic tool of global circulation. TEE allows us to study filling of the ventricles, contractility, the influence of the stabilizer, influence of dislocation of the right and left ventricle, pre-existing or induced valvular incompetence and quantification of vascular atherosclerosis.

Global examination at the beginning and end of the procedure include:

- *Global LV function:* assess what you are starting with prior to operation.
- *LV regional wall function:* note any or no abnormalities.
- *Estimate filling status of the heart.*
- *Mitral regurgitation (MR).*
- *RV function and tricuspid regurgitation (TR).*

- *Aortic valve:* check for regurgitation, calcification or abnormalities.
- *Aorta ascendens:* assess its health for any unidentified plaque in case of proximal anastomoses.

The value of TEE during the anastomotic period is of limited value. Evaluation of segmental regional wall motion abnormalities (SWMA's) during coronary clamping is cumbersome but may be indicative whether to use intracoronary shunts [17]. The persistence of SWMA's after OPCAB may be a predictor of complications during the immediate postoperative period [21]. Myocardial view is limited in the dislocated heart due to fixation and external pressure on the myocardium by the tissue stabilizer or other positioning devices. Since TEE distracts attention from the operative procedure, the investigation should be performed before cardiac manipulations. Another feature of TEE is the use of Doppler flow patterns. The use of pulmonary vein flow and transmitral flow gives valuable information about restrictive filling of the left ventricle and helps to identify beneficial effects of fluid loading, vasoactive medication or additional positioning devices such as the apical suction devices. It also allows control of graft flow after surgery [26] and is thus a form of indirect graft quality assessment.

▌ Cerebral monitoring

Monitoring cerebral blood flow by transcranial Doppler (TCD) is not part of standard monitoring. However, for research this is an important tool to investigate the impact of hemodynamics on cerebral oxygen metabolism and cerebral autoregulatory mechanisms. TCD may have a role not only in the detection of microemboli during manipulation of the aorta and during CPB but also as a monitor for cerebral hypoperfusion. TCD can identify the embolic load to the brain [28, 33]. This monitoring tool might give some answers to the question why cardiac surgery with CPB impairs cerebral function in some patients and how to change surgical strategies during surgery [2, 3, 5, 30]. For OPCAB patients considered at increased risk of adverse events concerning the central nervous system (CNS), direct monitoring of cerebral function may be indicated, particularly if episodic hypotension is anticipated. Use of the stroke risk index scale can aid in the selection of patients deemed at greatest CNS risk [23].

■ Temperature

Outcome of patients also depends on peri-operative temperature management. Patients (undergoing non-cardiac surgery) arriving in the ICU with a temperature < 35 °C have more ischemic cardiac complications [9, 10]. Maintaining normothermia reduces the risk of cardiac complications by 55% [10]. Hypothermia causes hypertension, tachycardia and an increase in catecholamine levels particularly in elderly patients. Hypothermia also shifts the oxygen dissociation curve to the left decreasing oxygen delivery to the tissues. Patients with postoperative myocardial ischemia have increased levels of cathecholamines during the operation and these increased levels correlate with a lower body temperature during the operation [1].

■ Assist devices during OPCAB

The question to assist or not by using hybrid perfusion techniques, modified myocardial tissue stabilizers or additional exposure instruments is difficult to answer. One should not forget that OPCAB has grown from a third world technique to a widespread accepted surgical technique in the western world. It allows coronary artery bypass surgery since the development of adequate tissue stabilizers. There are many centers performing almost all of the coronary cases as OPCAB. The results confirm that this technique is good if the surgical team is capable and each member of the team knows how to handle the specific problems faced during OPCAB surgery. To postulate that each operation will be better in terms of outcome when these assist devices are used, is not correct. Cost containment should remain an issue in this consideration. Investments into training of the surgeon and anesthesiologist has proven to be a better investment since almost 20% of the coronary bypass cases are performed by OPCAB worldwide and is still growing. The urge to use additional tools during OPCAB is also based on the fact that the procedure is more difficult than the conventional CABG with CPB, especially when initially using this technique. This applies for both the surgeon as the anesthesiologist.

Numerous positioning techniques and devices have been developed to facilitate access to target sites of coronary arteries during OPCAB. These include deep pericardial sutures (DPS), different patient positioning techniques, different surgical access techniques and various stabilizers. The hemodynamic effects may be reduced by specific maneuvers such as volume loading, deep Trendelenburg positioning [13], and cardiac herniation into a widely open right pleural space or the use of recently developed cardiac positioning devices like the Xpose™ Access Device (Guidant Corporation, Cupertino, USA) and the Starfish™ Access Device (Medtronic, Minneapolis, USA). They consist of a compliant suction cup, which conforms to the apex of the heart and is mounted to a sternal retractor via a multi-jointed, rigid shaft. These devices uncouple the function of positioning and stabilizing. By fixing the heart at two points (apex and base), the apical suction device itself provides a degree of target area stabilization prior to application of the stabilizer foot. By lifting the apex out of the chest, the apical suction device appears to elongate the collapsing left and right ventricular walls bringing the target area further out of the chest cavity and creating hemodynamic stability. These devices will help OPCAB procedures in certain cases [8, 29]. A balance between hemodynamic stability and cardiac manipulation in order to expose the target coronary anastomosis site, especially on the lateral and posterior wall, may still remain difficult in some cases. This hemodynamic compromise may result in the need for inotropic support or inadequate surgical view, which may lead to incomplete revascularization.

Aortic manipulation

Todate, most beating heart surgery operations are done as multi-vessel OPCAB procedures, which employ the use of a partial aortic clamp to perform proximal anastomoses. Yet the literature has repeatedly demonstrated that clamp application and removal is the greatest source of embolic activity during surgery and that the number of cerebral emboli is closely linked to subsequent adverse neurologic outcomes [3, 35]. A similar mechanism is likely during beating heart surgery, particularly since the partial aortic clamp is usually applied during maintenance of systemic mean arterial pressure. Until avoiding aortic instrumentation or partial aortic clamping is incorporated into beating heart procedures, it appears less likely that there will be significant improvements in overt neurological complications associated with multi-vessel revascularization. This concept has recently been provided by Calafiore and colleagues who reviewed their experiences with 4,875 patients undergoing either CABG or OPCAB with and without the use of a partial aortic clamp [6]. They demonstrated that in patients with extracoronary vasculopathy undergoing OPCAB procedures without evaluation of the ascending aorta, employment of aortic side-clamping was associated with the same CVA risk as observed in patients for whom CPB, aortic cannulation, and cross-clamping were used. Techniques designed to avoid use of the partial aortic occlusion clamp, especially in the absence of echographic evaluation of the ascending aorta, should be encouraged. One shot proximal staplers or devices avoiding aortic side-clamping are examples to be used but clinical results are awaited.

Conclusion

Since OPCAB has gained popularity as an alternative to CABG with CPB, strict attention to the details of planning and execution of beating heart procedures has become increasingly important. By avoiding right heart compression, hemodynamics can be preserved, thereby maintaining myocardial and systemic perfusion. Only when these objectives are met will OPCAB patients benefit from the potential advantages of the procedure. For OPCAB to be viable, graft patency rates must equal those achieved with arrested heart techniques. Maintenance of optimal hemodynamics, even in patients with impaired left ventricular function, can almost usually be achieved and will allow a precise, unhurried anastomosis under ideal conditions, maximizing the chance for successful revascularization.

References

1. Backlund M, Lepantalo M, Toivonen L, Tuominen M, Tarkkil P, Pere P, Scheinin M, Lindgren L (1999) Factors associated with post-operative myocardial ischaemia in elderly patients undergoing major non-cardiac surgery. Eur J Anaesthesiol 16:826–833
2. Barbut D, Lo YW, Hartman GS, Yao FS, Trifiletti RR, Hager DN, Hinton RB, Gold JP, Isom OW (1997) Aortic atheroma is related to outcome but not numbers of emboli during coronary bypass. Ann Thorac Surg 64:454–459
3. Barbut D, Yao FS, Hager DN, Kavanaugh P, Trifiletti RR, Gold JP (1996) Comparison of transcranial Doppler ultrasonography and transesophageal echocardiography to monitor emboli during coronary artery bypass surgery. Stroke 27:87–90
4. Boldt J, Hammermann H (1993) [The pulmonary artery catheter]. Anaesthesist 42:733–752
5. Borger MA, Taylor RL, Weisel RD, Kulkarni G, Benaroia M, Rao V, Cohen G, Fedorko L, Feindel CM (1999) Decreased cerebral emboli during distal aortic arch cannulation: a randomized clinical trial. J Thorac Cardiovasc Surg 118:740–745

6. Calafiore AM, Di Mauro M, Teodori G, Di Giammarco G, Cirmeni S, Contini M, Iaco AL, Pano M (2002) Impact of aortic manipulation on incidence of cerebrovascular accidents after surgical myocardial revascularization. Ann Thorac Surg 73:1387–1393

7. Cernaianu AC, DelRossi AJ, Boatman GA, Moore MW, Posner MA, Cilley JH Jr., Baldino WA, Santos ZL (1992) Continuous venous oximetry for hemodynamic and oxygen transport stability post cardiac surgery. J Cardiovasc Surg (Torino) 33:14–20

8. Dullum MK, Resano FG (2000) Xpose: a new device that provides reproducible and easy access for multivessel beating heart bypass grafting. Heart Surg Forum 3:113–117

9. Frank SM, Beattie C, Christopherson R, Norris EJ, Perler BA, Williams GM, Gottlieb SO (1993) Unintentional hypothermia is associated with postoperative myocardial ischemia. The Perioperative Ischemia Randomized Anesthesia Trial Study Group. Anesthesiology 78:468–476

10. Frank SM, Fleisher LA, Breslow MJ, Higgins MS, Olson KF, Kelly S, Beattie C (1997) Perioperative maintenance of normothermia reduces the incidence of morbid cardiac events. A randomized clinical trial. JAMA 277:1127–1134

11. Godje O, Thiel C, Lamm P, Reichenspurner H, Schmitz C, Schutz A, Reichart B (1999) Less invasive, continuous hemodynamic monitoring during minimally invasive coronary surgery. Ann Thorac Surg 68:1532–1536

12. Grundeman PF (1998) Vertical displacement of the beating heart by the Utrecht Octopus tissue stabilizer: effects on haemodynamics and coronary flow. Perfusion 13:229–230

13. Grundeman PF, Borst C, van Herwaarden JA, Mansvelt Beck HJ, Jansen EW (1997) Hemodynamic changes during displacement of the beating heart by the Utrecht Octopus method. Ann Thorac Surg 63:S88–S92

14. Grundeman PF, Borst C, Verlaan CW, Meijburg H, Moues CM, Jansen EW (1999) Exposure of circumflex branches in the tilted, beating porcine heart: echocardiographic evidence of right ventricular deformation and the effect of right or left heart bypass. J Thorac Cardiovasc Surg 118:316–323

15. Hamilton TT, Huber LM, Jessen ME (2002) Pulse CO: a less-invasive method to monitor cardiac output from arterial pressure after cardiac surgery. Ann Thorac Surg 74:S1408–S1412

16. London MJ, Moritz TE, Henderson WG, Sethi GK, O'Brien MM, Grunwald GK, Beckman CB, Shroyer AL, Grover FL (2002) Standard versus fiberoptic pulmonary artery catheterization for cardiac surgery in the Department of Veterans Affairs: a prospective, observational, multicenter analysis. Anesthesiology 96:860–870

17. Lucchetti V, Capasso F, Caputo M, Grimaldi G, Capece M, Brando G, Caprio S, Angelini GD (1999) Intracoronary shunt prevents left ventricular function impairment during beating heart coronary revascularization. Eur J Cardiothorac Surg 15:255–259

18. Mathison M, Buffolo E, Jatene AD, Jatene FB, Reichenspurner H, Matheny RG, Shennib H, Akin JJ, Mack MJ (2000) Right heart circulatory support facilities coronary artery bypass without cardiopulmonary bypass. Ann Thorac Surg 70:1083–1085

19. Mathison M, Edgerton JR, Horswell JL, Akin JJ, Mack MJ (2000) Analysis of hemodynamic changes during beating heart surgical procedures. Ann Thorac Surg 70:1355–1360

20. Mihaljevic T, von Segesser LK, Tonz M, Leskosek B, Seifert B, Jenni R, Turina M (1995) Continuous versus bolus thermodilution cardiac output measurements – a comparative study. Crit Care Med 23:944–949

21. Moises VA, Mesquita CB, Campos O, Andrade JL, Bocanegra J, Andrade JC, Buffolo E, Carvalho AC (1998) Importance of intraoperative transesophageal echocardiography during coronary artery surgery without cardiopulmonary bypass. J Am Soc Echocardiogr 11:1139–1144

22. Nelson LD (1986) Continuous venous oximetry in surgical patients. Ann Surg 203:329–333

23. Newman MF, Wolman R, Kanchuger M, Marschall K, Mora-Mangano C, Roach G, Smith LR, Aggarwal A, Nussmeier N, Herskowitz A, Mangano DT (1996) Multicenter preoperative stroke risk index for patients undergoing coronary artery bypass graft surgery. Multicenter Study of Perioperative Ischemia (McSPI) Research Group. Circulation 94:II74–II80

24. Nierich AP, Diephuis J, Jansen EW, Borst C, Knape JT (2000) Heart displacement during off-pump CABG: how well is it tolerated? Ann Thorac Surg 70:466–472

25. Nierich AP, Diephuis J, Jansen EW, van Dijk D, Lahpor JR, Borst C, Knape JT (1999) Embracing the heart: perioperative management of patients undergoing off-pump coronary artery bypass grafting using the octopus tissue stabilizer [see comments]. J Cardiothorac Vasc Anesth 13:123–129

26. Niimi Y, Morita S, Kaya K (1993) Intraoperative measurement of saphenous vein bypass graft flow with transesophageal echocardiography. J Cardiothorac Vasc Anesth 7:294–299

27. Odenstedt H, Stenqvist O, Lundin S (2002) Clinical evaluation of a partial CO_2 rebreathing technique for cardiac output monitoring in critically ill patients. Acta Anaesthesiol Scand 46:152–159

28. Pugsley W, Klinger L, Paschalis C, Treasure T, Harrison M, Newman S (1994) The impact of microemboli during cardiopulmonary bypass on neuropsychological functioning. Stroke 25:1393–1399

29. Sepic J, Wee JO, Soltesz EG, Hsin MK, Cohn LH, Laurence RG, Aklog L (2002) Cardiac positioning using an apical suction device maintains beating heart hemodynamics. Heart Surg Forum 5:279–284

30. Taylor RL, Borger MA, Weisel RD, Fedorko L, Feindel CM (1999) Cerebral microemboli during cardiopulmonary bypass: increased emboli during perfusionist interventions. Ann Thorac Surg 68:89–93

31. Thys DM (1996) Training, certification, and credentialing in transesophageal echocardiography. J Cardiothorac Vasc Anesth 10:309–310

32. van Aarnhem EE, Nierich AP, Jansen EW (1999) When and how to shunt the coronary circulation in off-pump coronary artery bypass grafting. Eur J Cardiothorac Surg 16 Suppl 2:S2–S6

33. van der Linden J, Casimir-Ahn H (1991) When do cerebral emboli appear during open heart operations? A transcranial Doppler study [see comments]. Ann Thorac Surg 51:237–241

34. Watters MP, Ascione R, Ryder IG, Ciulli F, Pitsis AA, Angelini GD (2001) Haemodynamic changes during beating heart coronary surgery with the 'Bristol Technique'. Eur J Cardiothorac Surg 19:34–40

35. Yao FS, Barbut D, Hager DN, Trifiletti RR, Gold JP (1996) Detection of aortic emboli by transesophageal echocardiography during coronary artery bypass surgery. J Cardiothorac Vasc Anesth 10:314–317

36. Yelderman M, Quinn MD, McKown RC, Eberhart RC, Dollar ML (1992) Continuous thermodilution cardiac output measurement in sheep. J Thorac Cardiovasc Surg 104:315–320

Anesthetic management

J. NICOLAI

Introduction

Beating heart cardiac surgery without cardiopulmonary bypass, also called off-pump coronary artery bypass (OPCAB) surgery, has gained more popularity in recent years. Even with limited evidence from prospective studies, published data suggest fewer complications normally associated with cardiopulmonary bypass (e.g., renal dysfunction, neurologic disorders, systemic inflammatory response syndromes) [2]. With the use of new technology like improved stabilizer and exposure systems, all sides of the heart can be reached and multivessel revascularization procedures can be performed. The surgical goals are summarized in Table 1 [6]. This increasing popularity has challenged the daily work of cardiovascular anesthesiologists. This article describes our approach to OPCAB procedures, the way we handle pitfalls and complications and may suggest a different attitude towards OPCAB surgery, always stressing the paramount subject: communication between anesthesiologist and surgeon.

Table 1. Cardiosurgical goals of OPCAB surgery [6]

- Less surgical trauma
- Reduction of morbidity and mortality
- Faster postoperative recovery
- Improvement of cost effectivity

Premedication and induction

All patients are seen the day before surgery, give written informed consent and receive an evening premedication of dikalium clorazepate of 20 mg p.o. Most patients are preoperatively treated with β-blockers and nitrates. This medication is continued up to the morning of surgery. In a case of severe hypertension we also continue prescribed ACE inhibitors. The morning premedication consists of dikalium clorazepate 20–40 mg p.o., 1 to 2 hours before surgery. After arrival in the induction room all patients are positioned on a water heated mattress and covered with a forced air warming blanket (Warm-Touch^{TM}). A pulse oximeter probe and a seven-channel ECG are applied, two leds, II/V5 are continuously displayed and used for ST-segment analysis. After local skin infiltration, we place a 14 gauge peripheral venous catheter and a 20 gauge radial artery catheter, preferable on the left hand side. General anesthesia is administered using 3–5 mg/kg of thiopentone, 5–8 µg/kg of fentanyl and 100 mg of suxamethonium. After the placement of a tracheal tube anesthesia is maintained using sevoflurane 1.5–3% in oxygen, fentanyl and rocoronium as muscle relaxants. We use sevoflurane because of the postulated preconditional and myocardial stabilizing effects and the good handling properties. We now insert a triple lumen central venous catheter in the right internal jugular vein. A gastric tube and a bladder catheter is placed, the later to monitor urine output and body temperature. To maintain body temperature, the Warm-Touch^{TM} blanket is used during the entire induction process.

Operation performance

In the operation room we ventilate the patient at a rate of 10 breaths per minute with a tidal volume of 8–10 ml/kg to keep the endtidal CO_2 level in the normal range. For patients undergoing endoscopic saphenous vein harvesting with CO_2 insufflation, we increase the respiration rate to overcome the potiential side effects of an elevated $ETCO_2$ [3]. After performing a median sternotomy and a incision of the pericardium, the surgeon dissects and prepares the left internal mammary artery (LIMA). If planned, the saphenous vein harvesting is performed simultaneously. With the completion of the LIMA harvesting, we administer 10,000 IU of heparin in order to achieve an activated coagulation time (ACT) of > 300 seconds. We do not use antifibrinolytic agents for OPCAB operations.

The crucial part of the operation, the OPCAB procedure itself, is the completion of the distal anastomosis of the coronary bypass. The anesthesiologist faces three major problems throughout this procedure [6]:

▌ Local cardiac motion is inhibited by the use of coronary stabilizing systems to enable a technically correct anastomosis.
▌ During the displacement of the heart, deterioration of cardiac function has to be minimized.
▌ Clamping of the respective coronary artery or branch may lead to regional ischemia and its complications.

To meet these challenges we follow a special perioperative protocol, which we established during recent years (see Table 2).

Before starting with the actual OPCAB procedure, the surgeon places a catheter in the left atrium for pressure monitoring (LAP). Then temporary epicardial pacemaker wires are sutured to the right atrium. The heart is paced at a rate of 90 beats per minute, suggesting that this is the optimal rate to achieve an optimal cardiac output [8]. A study at our clinic has shown that this procedure leads to superior cardiac stability, improves cardiac output by 25% and decreases stroke volume, left ventricle work load and consequently left ventricle oxygen consumption [4].

At our institution, we intend to start with the proximal anastomoses. Before the partial clamping of the aorta, the operating table is put in a steep anti-Trendelenburg position to lower the mean arterial pressure (MAP) to less than 60 mmHg. During

Table 2. Anesthetic management of OPCAB surgery (modified [5])

Hemodynamic stability during heart manipulation Reduction of myocardial ischemia Avoidance of arrhythmias	
Goals ▌ Ischemic tolerance ↑ ▌ Oxygen demand ↓ ▌ Oxygen supply ↑	**Procedures** ▌ Preconditioning ▌ Afterload control atrial pacing ▌ Nitrates **MAP** ↑ Intracoronary shunts
Monitoring ▌ LAP ▌ ECG ▌ TEE	

the completion of the proximal anastomoses, the anesthesiologist can precondition the patient's heart if necessary. We always infuse nitroglycerin at a rate of 1–2 mg/h to secure coronary artery dilatation. Most of the patients receive an Inzolen HK^{TM} infusion at a rate of 10–30 ml/h. Inzolen HK^{TM} is a mixed solution of potassium aspartate and magnesium aspartate with trace elements. This infusion is adminstered to maintain high normal potassium and magnesium levels, to prevent arrhythmia and to secure myocardial function during ischemia [7]. In a case of preoperatively impaired myocardial function (ejection fraction < 35%, high LAP even with atrial pacing), we consider an i.v. dose of enoximone 0.5–1 mg/kg. We use the positive inotropic properties without affecting the myocardial oxygen consumption, and thus avoiding catecholamine infusions. After finishing the proximal anastomoses, the ACT should still be above 300 s, if not we administer another 5000–10000 IU of heparin. Now the distal anastomoses are facilitated. In most of the cases the distal anatomosis to the circumflex artery and its branches

Table 3. Clinical grades of myocardial impairment

1. ST segment changes + stable MAP and LAP
2. LAP elevation + MAP deterioration
3. Ventricular arrhythmia

is performed first. The operation table is put in a steep Trendelenburg position and turned to the right. The surgeon mobilizes the heart. Deep pericardial sutures help to expose the lateral and posterior wall. Then the exposure device and the coronary stabilizer are placed to enable satisfactory suturing conditions. This has to be performed in a very cautious manner, in close communication and cooperation between surgeon and anesthesiologist. The hemodynamic situation has to be stable before proceeding with the operation. We always inform our surgical colleagues about the actual hemodynamic stability. We found three clinical grades of myocardial impairment that can occur during the course of the OPCAB procedure (see Table 3).

∎ Anesthetic actions

In a grade 1 situation, we may increase the nitroglycerin infusion and closely observe any further deterioration (Table 3).

In a grade 2 situation we would support the MAP with i.v. doses of diluted Akrinor^{TM}, a mixture of cafedrine and theoadrenaline, and i.v. fluids, if the MAP falls under 60 mmHg for a longer time. We would consider a change of the heart exposure or the positioning of the coronary stabilizer and the use of an intracoronary shunt, if not already in place.

A grade 3 situation is always a distinct warning to act immediately, because the next step would be ventricular tachycardia and subsequently defibrillation, and conversion to cardiopulmonary bypass is probably necessary. In such a situation, the surgeon has either to commence the anastomosis very quickly, if possible, or the heart has to be put back into the normal position and left resting there for some time, before we start another attempt in a different exposure or may continue with cardiopulmonary bypass.

Since we always use intracoronary shunts and atrial pacing during OPCAB procedures, we are in the fortunate position to experience such a situation very rarely. Our conversion rate to cardiopulmonary bypass is less than 1%.

Distal anastomoses to the LAD and the right coronary artery are facilitated in a similar manner, but used to be less demanding because the displacement of the heart is less extreme. After completion of all anastomoses, graft patency is assessed by using an ultrasound Doppler flow probe. When graft flow is satisfactory and hemodynamics are stable, protamine is administered at a 75% ratio of heparin used. When adequate hemotasis is obtained pericardium and sternum are closed. We take blood gas samples to verify good oxygenation and ventilation and to check a normal ACT. After skin closure, the patient is transferred to the intensive care unit (ICU). All patients are planned for a fast track recovery protocol, which means extubation within 2–4 hours and an ICU length of stay between 12 and 24 hours.

TEE

Since regional wall motion abnormalities (RWMA) are more sensitive indicators of myocardial ischemia than ECG changes, one can suggest that TEE monitoring should be the prime monitor during OPCAB operations. We do not use the TEE routinely, so our experience is limited. But direct vision of the exposed anterior and lateral wall allows an assessment of the respective coronary area. During procedures on the anterior wall, the transgastric short axial view, however, can be shown without greater difficulties and so regional wall motion abnormalities can be detected. During procedures on the posterior wall, the situation is different. Because of the displacement of the heart out of the pericardial cavity, it is very difficult if not impossible to obtain a reasonable accurate TEE view.

But there might be another indication for TEE examination during OPCAB surgery. It can be useful to assess the left ventricle, especially if it has been examined as poor previously, evaluate ejection fraction and RWMA, immediately prior the OPCAB procedure itself, to initiate preconditioning if necessary.

Temperature control management

As previously said, it is very important to preserve a normal body temperature. We start with temperature conversation in the induction room, because it is very difficult to regain lost body temperature during the operation. As mentioned earlier, we use a WarmTouch^{TM} blanket and prewarmed fluids. In the operation room we raise room temperature up to 24–26 °C, heat the water mattress to 38–39 °C and perform a low-flow anesthetic with a fresh gas flow of not more than 1 l/min if possible. When there is no venous grafting planned, we can keep the forced air warming blanket on the lower half of the patient. So we are able to maintain a body temperature above 36 °C in most of our patients, regardless the number of grafts necessary. In the rare case of a lower body temperature, the WarmTouch^{TM} blanket can be used in the ICU postoperatively as well.

Fluid management

To maintain a good venous filling more i.v. fluids have to be administered during OPCAB procedures compared to on pump coronary artery bypass surgery. We always use warmed fluids on a cristalloid/colloid ratio of 2:1. We use Ringer-lactate solution as the cristalloid and 6% of hetastarch as the colloid fluid. During the course of the operation, we give an adequate amount of volume to achieve a urine output of 1 ml/kg/h, normally between 2 and 3 L. We consider a hematocrit of 24–25% as a threshold for blood transfusion. We would not use a cell saver for a routine case, because we have found out that it is economical only in selected cases.

Prospects

Recent studies of OPCAB surgery suggest an ultra fast track anesthetic technique, using general anesthesia and thoracic epidural analgesia, leading to early extubation and discharge from the ICU. Further evaluation needs to be done, whether this might be a way to earlier hospital discharge, better outcome, more cost saving and greater patient contentment [1].

Conclusion

Throughout the last few years, we have increased our knowledge about cardiac pathophysiology and our experience about OPCAB procedures, through the regular work with this operation technique. This expertise, a strict anesthetic protocol and the cooperation with our surgical colleagues, disapproved our partial prejudices and encouraged us to proceed with OPCAB operations.

We now perform this operation on a regular basis and we assume that it will result in less invasive and more cost-effective coronary artery bypass surgery.

Summary

Off-pump coronary artery bypass grafting (OPCAB) has gained more popularity for bypass surgery in recent years. To face the anesthesiologic challenge we have established a perioperative protocol. This protocol consists of adequate fluid mangement, temperature control mangement and increased intraoperative monitoring (arterial, centralvenous and left atrial pressure, five-channel ECG). To mantain sufficent cardiac output during the OPCAB procedure, we use atrial pacing and initiate optimal venous filling. However good communication between surgeon and anesthesiologist is the main factor to achieve successful results in OPCAB surgery and better patient outcome.

References

1. Djaiani GN, Ali M, Heinrich L, Bruce J, Carroll J, Karski J, Cusimano RJ, Cheng DCH (2001) Ultra-fast-track anesthetic technique facilitates operating room extubation in patients undergoing off-pump coronary revascularization surgery. J Cardiothorac Vasc Anesth 15:152–157
2. Eldrup N, Rasmussen NH, Yndgaard S, Bigler D, Berthelsen PG (2001) Impact of off-pump coronary artery surgery on myocardial performances and β-adrenoceptor function. J Cardiothorac Vasc Anesth 15:428–432
3. Gaynes JM (1999) The minimally invasive cardiac surgery voyage. J Cardiothorac Vasc Anesth 13:119–122
4. Gulielmos V, Kappert U, Nicolai J, Eller M, Sahre H, Alexiou K, Georgi C, Hartmann N (2002) Improving hemodynamics during off-pump bypass surgery by atrial pacing. The Heart Surgery Forum (in press)
5. Kessler P, Lischke V, Westphal K (2000) Anäshesiologische Besonderheiten bei minimalinvasiver Herzchirurgie. Anaesthesist 49:592–608
6. Nierich AP, Diephuis J, Jansen EWL, van Dijk D, Lahpor JR, Borst C, Knape JTA (1999) Embracing the heart: perioperative manage-

ment of patients undergoing off-pump coronary artery bypass grafting using the octopus stabilizer. J Cardiothorac Vasc Anesth 13:123–
129
7. Schroll A (2000) Intensivtherapie mit INZOLEN®. Innovations-Ver-
   lags-Gesellschaft m.b.H., Seeheim-Jugenheim, pp 43–64
8. Sowton E (1964) Hemodynamic studies in patients with artificial
   pacemakers. Brit Heart J 26:737–746

Atrial stimulation during OPCAB

A simple maneuver to maintain stable hemodynamics during OPCAB

V. Gulielmos, U. Kappert, M. Eller, H. Sahre

Introduction

Off-pump surgery is proposed to avoid inflammatory response, renal and pulmonary, but above all thromboembolic episodes [1, 6–8]. Even if most cardiac surgeons acknowledge the advantages of a cardiac procedure avoiding cardiopulmonary bypass, very few have changed their surgical concept to OPCAB. The main reason for that is the hemodynamic instability occurring while tilting the heart, mostly for exposure of the back wall vessels of the left ventricle.

Among the maneuvers proposed for better tolerance of displacing the heart for beating heart procedures, like the Trendelenburg maneuver, right rotation of the operating table [2, 3], or the "Lima stitch", is temporary atrial pacing.

Technique and comment

After a median sternotomy is performed, the pericardium is opened and temporary pacemaker wires are sutured epicardially with interrupted sutures (5-0 prolene). Atrial pacing is then started with a pacing frequency of 90 per minute. The positive hemodynamic effect of the maneuver is then immediately acknowledged by immediate increase of systolic (RRs) and mean arterial pressure (RRm), whereas left atrial (LAP) and central venous pressure (CVP) significantly decrease. In parallel and as shown in a clinical study at our institution a significant increase of cardiac output (CO) and cardiac index (CI) is observed [4].

Most patients suffering from coronary artery disease are on β-blockers and therefore appear with normo- to rather brady-cardia at admission to hospital. The negative chronotropic effects of this medication becomes more evident when sedation drugs for general anesthesia are applied [4]. The patient's heart rate is then paced up to 90 per minute.

At that point the question rises why 90 per minute. Sawton et al. have shown very clearly already in the 1970s that the human heart performance with regards to CO and CI reaches its maximum around this frequency at rest [5]. It is no wonder then why arterial pressure also rises. This is the first positive effect of the proposed maneuver, because most cardiac surgeons performing OPCAB realize that RR decreases when the heart is displaced.

In addition to the increase of RR, the positive effects of atrial pacing are appreciated by further stabilization of the left ventricular performance.

While tilting of the heart for exposure of the back wall coronary vessels, the left ventricle is pressed against the pericardium, consisting in deformation of left ventricular geometry, decreasing LV function and decreasing RR sometimes necessitating conversion to CPB.

Atrial pacing leads to a decrease of stroke volume [4] meaning that the radius of the chamber of the left ventricle is also decreased (Fig. 1). The law of LaPlace taught us that wall stress is proportional to the radius of the chamber, meaning that with a decrease of the chamber radius (in this case the radius of the left ventricle), the wall stress also decreases. Since the wall stress of the left ventricle is decreased the contracting condition of the left ventricle is more stable, meaning that tilting the heart is tolerated far better, consisting of more stable hemodynamics.

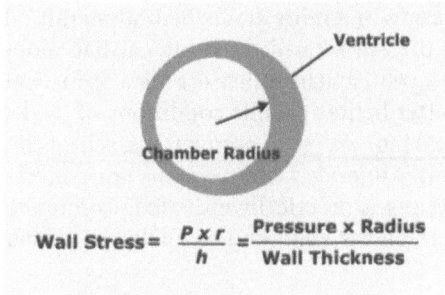

Fig. 1. Law of La Place: if pressure or radius increase, wall stress increases

In case of a functionally mitral valve regurgitation, left ventricular performance is also set under pressure. If an OPCAB procedure is scheduled the Trendelenburg maneuver is not well tolerated, in that particular case, due to the additional left ventricular volume load. When atrial pacing is performed, a decrease of stroke volume and, thus, a decrease of the left ventricular chamber radius occurs. In addition to correction of electrical atrial-ventricular interval, compitance of the mitral valve occurs, consisting in better tolerance of the additional volume load during the Trendelenburg maneuver.

The described maneuver is routinely used in our OPCAB cases, thus sparing the procedures from hemodynamic deterioration while tilting the heart and conversion to CPB is practically deleted.

Summary

For a safer hemodynamic situation during OPCAB procedures, several maneuvers were proposed including the Trendelenburg position or right rotation of the operating table. Temporary atrial stimulation was proved to increase ventricular performance consisting in a more stable hemodynamic situation regarding arterial pressure, cardiac output, cardiac index, but also by decreasing left ventricular wall stress via a reduction in its radius. Due to the better hemodynamic conditions of the left ventricle, tilting of the heart for access of coronary vessels of the back wall of the heart is better tolerated and necessity for conversion to cardiopulmonary bypass is practically excluded. Combination of the above maneuvers allows solid and safe OPCAB surgery.

References

1. Ascione R, Lloyd CT, Underwood MJ, Gomes WJ, Angelini GD (1999) On-pump versus off-pump coronary revascularization: evaluation of renal function. Ann Thorac Surg 68:493–498
2. Benetti FJ, Ballester C, Sani G, Boonstra P, Grandjean J (1995) Video assisted coronary bypass surgery. J Card Surg 10:620–625
3. Gruendemann PF, Borst C, Verlaan CWJ, Meijburg H, Mouës, Jansen EWL (1999) Exposure of circumflex branches in the tilted, beating porcine heart: echocardiographic evidence of right ventricular deformation and the effect of right or left heart bypass. J Thorac Cardiov Sur 118:316–323
4. Gulielmos V, Kappert U, Eller M, Sahre H, Alexiou K, Georgi C, Nicolai J, Hartmann N (2003) Improving hemodynamics during off-pump bypass surgery by atrial pacing. Heart Surg Forum (in press)
5. Sowton E (1964) Hemodynamic studies in patients with artificial pacemakers. Brit Heart J 26:737–746
6. Strüber M, Cremer JT, Gohrbandt B, Hagl C, Jankowski M, Völker B, Rückoldt H, Martin M, Haverich A (1999) Humane cytokine responses to coronary artery bypass grafting with and without cardiopulmonary bypass. Ann Thorac Surg 68:1330–1335
7. Trehan N, Mishra M, Sharma OP, Mishra A, Kasliwal RR (2001) Further reduction in stroke after off-pump coronary artery bypass grafting: a 10-year experience. Ann Thorac Surg 72:1026–1032
8. Wan S, Izzat MB, Lee TW, Wan IYP, Tang NLS, Yim APC (1999) Avoiding cardiopulmonary bypass in multivessel CABG reduces cytokine response and myocardial injury. Ann Thorac Surg 68:52–57

Developing on OPCAB program

I. Friedrich, J. Börgermann

Summary

Developing an OPCAB program needs good preparation prior to performing the first operation. Visiting a high volume program is highly recommended. A step by step approach to OPCAB surgery, beginning with revascularization of the anterior wall, might reduce the hazards of this technique and allows both the surgeon and the anesthesiologist to become familiar with this technique.

Being convinced

Why should one depart from a proven technique that has been successfully used for decades and that was shown to have a reproducibly low complication rate, and suddenly favor a technically much more demanding method?

Prospective randomized studies which are now available have proven the advantages of the OPCAB approach [2, 15]. OPCAB can prevent life-threatening and debilitating complications, especially in patients with specific risk factors, such as severe calcification of the ascending aorta.

Recent prospective studies were instrumental in showing advantages of OPCAB compared to the conventional approach. By performing a diligent analysis of the literature and by attending conferences related to the topic, interested surgeons can collect the information required for starting an OPCAB program and for discussing the changeover with both the referring cardiologists and the surgical team. Only surgeons convinced that OPCAB has considerable advantages compared to the conventional approach can carry this motivation into their surgical teams [9]. Involving the referring cardiologists at the earliest stages of establishing an OPCAB program and explaining the scientific basis behind the approach are certainly sensible preliminary steps. It is known from experience that most cardiological colleagues gladly accept less invasive approaches. But it is the surgeon who has to provide the impetus for the change. Willingness to depart from a reliable technique in favor of something completely new is mandatory. When doing OPCAB procedures, the surgeon's sensibility, flexibility, and communication skills are highly challenged. Strict adherence to a pre-defined straightforward sequence is often impossible. The outcome of an OPCAB procedure frequently depends on the surgeon's ability to adjust to the specific intraoperative conditions and to match the procedural details to the particular hemodynamic state after prior consultation with the anesthesiologist.

Involving the team

For the anesthesiologist, the required changes are even greater than for the surgeon. While anesthesiologists used to have to pay most attention to weaning from extracorporeal circulation (ECC), they now (in beating heart surgery) have to be involved in each surgical step. The anesthesiological colleagues should therefore be part of any plans to establish an OPCAB program, preferably during the earliest phases. *Joint* trips to centers with extensive experience are essential for the successful launch of an OPCAB program. Anesthesiologists, surgeons, and, if possible, OR nursing staff should participate. The observed surgical steps and anesthesiological techniques should be documented during these visits. It seems helpful to initially emulate the techniques used at the center which appears to have the most comprehensible approach. With growing experience, the initially chosen techniques can be modified and adapted to one's individual needs. The OR nursing staff also needs to be involved in the early stages of planning an OPCAB program. Specific differences to the conventional technique, the sequence of operative events including the most critical phases, and handling of additional instruments should be taught in specialized training seminars conducted long before the first procedure is scheduled. The availability of specific instruments, such as stabilizers, snares and shunts needs to be ascertained by the surgeon prior to conducting the first procedures. In addition, technical prerequisites (adequate suction, cellsaver, and availability of a suitable CO_2 source for the blower/mister) have to be taken care of. For OPCAB procedures, the perfusionists are primarily concerned with technical devices such as cellsavers and suction units. Perfusionists are therefore still tied into the course of the operation. One needs to categorically counter any impression that perfusionists are redundant for OPCAB procedures. Their presence in the operating room is indispensable for the safe conduct of OPCAB procedures, and perfusionists continue to be indispensable members of the surgical team.

Trusting each other

There is hardly another surgical procedure that requires such close cooperation between surgeon and anesthesiologist as OPCAB. Without a strong bond of trust between anesthesiologist and surgeon, OPCAB surgery is doomed to fail. After establishing adequate exposure, the surgeon will fully concentrate on quickly completing a perfect peripheral anastomosis. The anesthesiologist should be able to estimate the time required by the surgeon, in order to request conversion to ECC at just the proper time in case the patient's hemodynamics deteriorate. Meeting such a request without discussion and in a timely manner is essential for the survival of the entire OPCAB program. Converting too early is not associated with any specific risks, but converting too late can have lethal results [13]. In order to make a positive experience, the anesthesiologist needs to be sure that his/her request for conversion will be accepted as a responsible decision. With increasing confidence, the anesthesiologist can begin to explore the limits and learn how to control more difficult situations. With growing experience, all centers with great OPCAB case numbers see a steadily decreasing conversion rate.

Becoming familiar with the technique

Performing the first cases with ECC support on the beating heart is a sensible approach for becoming familiar with the various commercial stabilizing devices. One should do the first OPCAB cases in patients who fulfill most of the criteria listed in Table 1. Even if high-risk patients are likely to profit most from the OPCAB technique, at the beginning of an OPCAB program one should start with patients whose operative risk is low. Going through a so-called learning curve with initially marginal results

Table 1. Initial patient selection when starting an off-pump program

▮ Good LV function

▮ Hemodynamic stability

▮ Good caliber coronary arteries with a superficial course

▮ No myocardial hypertrophy

▮ No COPD

is unacceptable and can only be avoided by exercising extreme caution [11]. Initially, one should limit oneself to revascularization of the anterior wall and proximal RCA. After a sufficient number of OPCAB cases (50–100), one can expand the indications to include the patient population that derives the most benefit from this technique. The elderly, patients with reduced LV function, patients with prior neurological diseases, and patients in whom multiple organ systems are impaired appear to derive a more than proportional profit from the OPCAB approach [1, 5, 10, 14]. IABP support should be considered in patients with severely reduced LV function and should be used in most patients with acute myocardial infarction.

The transition from the conventional to the OPCAB technique should be gradual. Any problems or complications encountered should be analyzed after each respective case.

Succeeding

Being able to reflect critically is one of the essentials for success when starting with any new technique. That includes the willingness to subject one's own work to exacting quality control standards. When first starting with OPCAB surgery, it is sensible and necessary to perform postoperative cardiac catheterization and coronary angiography to visualize the anastomoses [3, 6]. This type of quality control is particularly meaningful for the surgeon, but also for the entire surgical team. It also proves to the cardiological colleagues that the surgical technique is successful. In an established and successful program, training and continuing training in OPCAB are unproblematic. In some hospitals, cardiac surgical residents have performed all their coronary revascularization procedures with the OPCAB technique. Several studies demonstrate that training surgeons in OPCAB surgery does not expose patients to an increased risk [4, 8, 12]. Simulators could make sense when training surgeons, but they have not yet found widespread acceptance [7]. In a large number of working groups, the OPCAB frequency is close to 100%, but this cannot be the goal in each department. Organizational aspects have to be considered when determining the desirable and achievable share of OPCAB procedures in a cardiac surgical department. The potential OPCAB benefit needs to be realistically weighed against the potential risk. In some hospitals, the core cardiac surgical anesthesiologists are not necessarily always available during on-call hours. It may therefore not always be sensible to use OPCAB in emergency cases when the team is comprised of staff members mostly inexperienced in OPCAB.

Most often, individual surgeons will take the initiative to explore the new method. These individuals should then train interested team members in OPCAB. These team members can act as multipliers. No surgeon or anesthesiologist should be forced to use the technique; otherwise the results would probably be worse than if the staff members had stuck to conventional surgery. Motivation and a positive attitude are essential requirements for good surgical results.

Seven maxims for surgeons

▌ Talk to your anesthesiologists.
▌ Use shunts if possible.
▌ Don't rush.
▌ Check graft flow (flow meter).
▌ Consider IABP in cases of acute myocardial infarction and/or when the ventricle is bad.
▌ Conversion is not a catastrophe, but prevents a catastrophe.
▌ Not every surgeon or anesthesiologist will be comfortable with OPCAB.

References

1. Akpinar B, Guden M, Sanisoglu I, Sagbas E, Caynak B, Bayramoglu Z et al (2001) Does off-pump coronary artery bypass surgery
   reduce mortality in high risk patients? Heart Surg Forum 4(3):
   231–236
2. Angelini GD, Taylor FC, Reeves BC, Ascione R (2002) Early and
   midterm outcome after off-pump and on-pump surgery in Beating
   Heart Against Cardioplegic Arrest Studies (BHACAS 1 and 2): a
   pooled analysis of two randomised controlled trials. Lancet
   359(9313):1194–1199
3. Bergsland J, D'Ancona G, Karamanoukian H, Ricci M, Schmid S,
   Salerno TA (2000) Technical tips and pitfalls in OPCAB surgery:
   the Buffalo experience. Heart Surg Forum 3(3):189–193
4. Burack J (2001) Resident training in off-pump CABG. Ann Thorac
   Surg 71(1):398–399
5. Chamberlain MH, Ascione R, Reeves BC, Angelini GD (2002) Evaluation of the effectiveness of off-pump coronary artery bypass
   grafting in high-risk patients: an observational study. Ann Thorac
   Surg 73(6):1866–1873
6. D'Ancona G, Karamanoukian HL, Salerno TA, Schmid S, Bergsland
   J (1999) Flow measurement in coronary surgery. Heart Surg Forum
   2(2):121–124
7. Izzat MB, El-Zufari MH, Yim AP (1998) Training model for "beating-heart" coronary artery anastomoses. Ann Thorac Surg 66(2):
   580–581
8. Karamanoukian HL, Panos AL, Bergsland J, Salerno TA (2000)
   Perspectives of a cardiac surgery resident in-training on off-pump
   coronary bypass operation. Ann Thorac Surg 69(1):42–5; discussion 45–46
9. Masroor S, Salerno T (2002) How to start a beating heart coronary
   artery surgery program. The Heart Surgery Forum 5(3):237–239
10. Meharwal ZS, Trehan N (2002) Off-pump coronary artery bypass
    grafting in patients with left ventricular dysfunction. Heart Surg
    Forum 5(1):41–45
11. Novick RJ, Fox SA, Stitt LW, Swinamer SA, Lehnhardt KR, Rayman
    R et al (2001) Cumulative sum failure analysis of a policy change
    from on-pump to off-pump coronary artery bypass grafting. Ann
    Thorac Surg 72(3):1016–1021

12. Ricci M, Karamanoukian HL, D'Ancona G, DeLaRosa J, Karama-noukian RL, Choi S et al (2000) Survey of resident training in beating heart operations. Ann Thorac Surg 70(2):479–482
13. Soltoski P, Salerno T, Levinsky L, Schmid S, Hasnain S, Diesfeld T et al (1998) Conversion to cardiopulmonary bypass in off-pump coronary artery bypass grafting: its effect on outcome. J Card Surg 13(5):328–334
14. Trehan N, Mishra M, Kasliwal RR, Mishra A (2000) Surgical strate-gies in patients at high risk for stroke undergoing coronary artery bypass grafting. Ann Thorac Surg 70(3):1037–1045
15. van Dijk D, Nierich AP, Jansen EW, Nathoe HM, Suyker WJ, Diephuis JC et al (2001) Early outcome after off-pump versus on-pump coronary bypass surgery: results from a randomized study. Circulation 104(15):1761–1766

Surgical technique for off-pump coronary artery bypass grafting

V. Gulielmos, U. Kappert, M. Eller, H. Sahre,
K. Alexiou, C. Georgi, J. Nicolai

Introduction

The first attempts for developing an extracorporeal circulation system are found at the beginning of the 20th century, performed by so-called heart and circulation physiologists, with the aim of gaining access to the interior of the heart. Even if coronary artery bypass grafting is performed on the surface of the heart and initial procedures were performed without the use of cardiopulmonary bypass [6], the spread of use of cardiopulmonary bypass in cardiac surgery has led cardiac surgeons to always use the heart lung machine, even in bypass procedures. The median sternotomy played an important role, as it gives excellent access to the great vessels and enables easy and safe cannulation for extracorporeal circulation. On the other hand, the use of the heart lung machine enabled easier access to all coronary vessels with stable hemodynamics, in addition to ideal immobilization of coronary arteries. The above presented concept consisting of median sternotomy plus cardiopulmonary bypass (CPB) has been used for the past four decades. Cardiac surgery was very convenient for cardiac surgeons, who did not have to think about the kind of surgical access nor about the use of CPB or not. In the mid 1990s new procedures were presented changing this concept [1–3, 5, 8, 9]. Coronary artery bypass grafting without the use of CPB was, however, used previously in developing countries due to commercial aspects.

The first standardized OPCAB procedure was developed by an experimental cardiologist and included the Octopus device [2]. We adapted the off-pump technique at our institution in 1996 and started performing CABG without CPB mostly in patients with exclusion criteria for CPB, such as low left ventricular ejection fraction (LVEF), impaired lung and renal function, peripheral vascular disease, and cerebral vascular insufficiency. This means that even though we were not experienced in OP-CAB surgery, we rather reserved this technique mostly for heavily diseased patients. After almost a year we realized that for safe use of off-pump technique greater experience was necessary. Off-pump procedures were then used more often in patients with suitable coronary morphology meaning that this technique was reserved for patients necessitating grafting of the anterior left ventricular wall and of the right coronary artery being easier accessible. By exchanging the device with a more mature coronary artery stabilizer, the incidence of off-pump surgery increased at our institution. As exposing systems (Xpose Guidant, Santa Clara, CA; Starfish™, Medtronic, Minneapolis, MN) came on the market, exposure of coronaries of the back wall of the left ventricle became easier and grafts per patient increased with a lower conversion rate to CPB. With time and by gaining more experience by introducing mature coronary stabilizing and exposing devices, further development of the anesthesia protocol, exposing technique, and anastomotic technique quality of anastomoses increased and anastomotic complications decreased. In the following we present a mature OPCAB technique practically excluding the necessity of conversion to CPB and offering a very low rate of anastomotic complications.

Surgical technique and comment

The patient is placed in the supine position and under general anesthesia. After the left IMA and additional arterial or vein grafts are harvested the pericardium is opened longitudinally in the shape of reversed "T" at its diaphragmal aspects. Using an OPCAB retractor (CTS, Guidant, Santa Clara, CA), we use 4 pericardial stay sutures incising the right distal pericardium at its diaphragmatic aspects towards the inferior cava vein. This maneuver is used if the right IMA is not harvested and the right pleura remains closed. It enables displacing of the heart more into the right pleura while exposing obtuse marginal (OM) vessels, either of the circumflex or of the right coronary system. After incising the pericardium, a left atrial catheter is inserted via the right superior pulmonary vein into the left atrium for continuous left atrial pressure (LAP) monitoring. Epicardial pacemaker wires are sutured at the appendage of the right atrium for atrial stimulation for improving hemodynamics [4]. Monitoring of LAP in addition to mean arterial pressure helps to estimate volume load and left ventricular performance concurrently. The anesthesiologist has time to precondition the left ventricle using nitroglycerine or in rare cases additionally enoximone if LAP is very high and mean arterial pressure is low [7]. Going on with the surgical procedure, proximal anastomoses are performed first. In case of aortic proximal anastomoses, a side biting clamp is placed performing an anti-"Trendelenburg" maneuver in order to further decrease arterial pressure and to "smoothen" the ascending aorta. This also gives the surgeon the opportunity to estimate the degree of calcification of the ascending aorta and to decide to attach proximal anastomoses to the aorta or not. In case of use of multiple arterial conduits, Y-grafts are performed between the LIMA and other arterial conduits (RIMA, radial artery etc.). Proximal anastomoses are always performed in a continuous over-and-over manner using a 6.0 Prolene between aorta and veins and 7.0 Prolene for other arterial conduits. We do not start coronary anastomoses by LIMA to LAD as previously proposed to immediately perfuse the anterior wall and diaphragm. We believe that as the heart is beating without the attached bypass at least at rest (anesthesia) this is not necessary. We generally start with the obtuse marginal branches from the right, then from the circumflex moving to the intermediates, diagonals, LAD, and at the end we graft the right or the PDA. That way the target coronary vessels move in one way counter clockwise. For exposure of the posterolateral wall of the left ventricle, we perform the Trendelenburg maneuver and rotate the table to the right in order to always have enough volume load of the heart and additionally to allow the left ventricle to move towards the right pleura. Using a deep pericardial stitch to the left posterior junction of the pericardium to the diaphragm, we also tilt the heart to the right. The use of an exposing device enables pulling and stretching of the heart into its longitudinal axis and displacing it even more to the right for better exposure of the OM system. Pulling the heart in its longitudinal axis decreases the transverse radius of the heart. The Law of La-Place taught us that with decreasing radius of the chamber also decreases wall stress of the chamber, resulting in this particular case in better tolerance of heart displacement. After exposure of the coronary vessels a coronary stabilizing system using the combination of suction and pressure (Axius^{TM}, Guidant, Santa Clara, CA) is used for coronary stabilization. A segment of the coronary artery is free dissected. In case that the segment is not suitable for insertion of an anastomosis a more suitable segment of the coronary artery is sought. After the segment of the coronary artery is found for insertion of coronary anastomosis, a tourniquet is passed directly proximal around the vessel for temporary coronary occlusion, but is not yet snared. The length of the conduit is measured by placing the graft across the circumflex artery and across the OM and its distal end is prepared for the anastomosis. Before occlusion of the coronary artery using the snare and with a small sharp blade the coronary is opened while it is still perfused. This always leads to bleeding, but avoids hurting the back wall as the diameter of the coronary artery is maximal due to the perfused vessel. The proximal snare is then used to control bleeding. Using a pair of potts scissors, a coronarotomy is completed. We generally perform longer anastomoses, approximately 6 to 8 mm. Anastomoses are longer for vein grafts than for arterial grafts, because the longer the coronary anastomosis is the smaller the possibility for twisting the conduit close to the anastomosis. A coronary shunt is always used. The diameter of the shunt is chosen depending on the diameter of the coronary artery. Even in proximal occluded coronary arteries a shunt is inserted as we have faced in the past myocardial ischemia during coronary occlusion, even in proximally occluded coronary vessels. The reason why we do not wait to use the coronary shunt until ischemia has occurred, has to do with the fact that insertion of a coronary shunt is not always as easy. If the surgeon needs a longer time for insertion of the coronary shunt, this might lead to non-reversible myocardial ischemia when dealing with low ejection fraction ventricles. However, in case that a surgeon feels that coronary shunts should not be used, we have determined in our initial off-pump practice that ischemia signs on ECG in terms of ST elevation are not an indication for use of a shunt. We found that more important warning ischemia signs leading to left ventricular decompensation include arrhythmia, severe decrease of blood pressure or severe increase of LAP. The anastomosis is then started with a parachuting technique starting at the heel and using a continuous over-and-over suture (7.0 Prolene). Before the last one or two stitches of the anastomosis, the shunt is removed and bleeding is controlled by pulling at the suture. Before tying the knots the proximal snare suture is completely removed first in order to allow probe insertion first distally and then proximally. This maneuver does not seem to hurt the intima as the coronary artery is perfused and normothermic. On the other hand, if due to the shunt insertion the intima is damaged the probe would even straighten it. During this maneuver, the anastomosis bleeds antegradely and retrogradely. This flush maneuver helps to wash small particles (debris) from the anastomosis. This would not happen if cardioplegic arrest had been used. Also before tying the knots of the suture of the anastomosis the bulldog of the conduit is removed and an additional flush maneuver through the conduit is performed in an antegrade fashion for the same reason. This is also the reason why we believe that the more calcified the coronary vessel is the better it is for the patient to be operated off-pump. With cardioplegic arrest, debris (small particles) is released by stitching through the plaque, which remains within the anastomosis. After tying the knots of the suture and while testing the anastomosis by injecting through the conduit into the coronary vessel, this debris would flow into the coronary artery thus causing myocardial microembolisms. Using the presented OPCAB anastomotic technique this complication is totally excluded. This can be appreciated at our institution by the seldomly observed ischemia signs on ECG and no increase of cardiac enzymes in our off-pump procedures. After the anastomosis is performed the coronary stabilizing device is removed and the next coronary artery is stabilized. We always perform flow measurement of our bypass grafts using Doppler sonography. However, the total flow per minute through the bypass is not as important as the graphic applied. In case that flow is insufficient and ischemia signs on ECG occur we always revise the anastomosis. The use of a shunt generally excludes the case of anastomotic complication; however, if in very small vessels a shunt can not be used due to the small diameter of the vessel, the potential of the coronary anastomosis complication is present. A potential complication is stitching through the shunt or through the suture of the shunt. Such complications occurred previously and they were managed by cutting the plastic of the shunt or the suture of the shunt. Extremely seldom we have to redo the anastomosis because of damage to the anastomotic suture.

Using coronary shunts, coronary anastomoses are more demanding, e.g., in the past the anastomotic times were 4.0 minutes/anastomosis and using the shunts the anastomotic time increased to 7.4 minutes/anastomosis. However, as the coronary artery is continuously perfused the surgeon has time to perform the anastomosis.

The impact of this anastomotic technique can be appreciated by the fact that only one conversion to CPB during the last 430 off-pump procedures was necessary at our institution. In this particular case with occluded LAD and right coronary artery on a low ejection fraction ventricle (LVEF = 25%), the only coronary artery perfusing practically the whole myocardium was a 70% stenosed circumflex artery. The vessel was occluded and prepared for insertion of a shunt while accidentally the suction of both devices, exposing and stabilizing devices, was switched off. The tilted heart fell into the pericardium. Before again exposing and stabilizing the coronary artery in order to insert the shunt, the low ejection fraction ventricle became hypoxemic and conversion to CPB was necessary. This patient received a triple graft procedure and was weaned from CPB with the support of an intraaortic balloon pump without inotropic support and left the hospital on postoperative day 8.

Hemodynamic or arrhythmia complications on ICU only occurred 4 times. An 84-year old lady receiving 4 grafts was extubated and had ventricular fibrillation three hours postoperatively. After electrical defibrillation, the patient's hemodynamics was stabilized immediately and the patient did not need reintubation. Although cardiac enzymes remained negative and no ischemia signs on ECG occurred the patient received a control angiography revealing excellent patency of all 4 anastomoses. The explanation for fibrillation was a hypertonic crisis just before ventricular fibrillation of the old hypertrophic ventricle.

In a further patient, severe decrease of arterial pressure occurred, leading to resuscitation on ICU 2 hours after operation. After the patient was stabilized grafts were controlled by angiogram revealing all 3 anastomoses to have excellent patency. The decrease of the arterial pressure in this particular patient was explained by the use of sedation. The patient was discharged on postoperative day 6 from the hospital.

Another patient revealed 4 hours postoperatively ischemia signs on ECG and necessitated inotropic support. The patient was brought to the cath lab and coronary angiography revealed excellent patency of all 3 anastomoses with a LAD occlusion

5 mm distally to the insertion of the LIMA to the LAD. The LAD underwent PTCA and was stented, however, with a moderate result and the decision was made for additional distal bypass grafting on the LAD. The procedure was also performed off-pump, as the patient was then completely hemodynamically stable, not necessitating any inotropic support or the intraaortic balloon pump. The patient had an uneventful second procedure, but died on postoperative day 16 due to pneumonia. In this particular patient a coronary shunt was used for the LIMA to LAD anastomosis, as the LAD was heavily calcified not being able to be occluded using snares. However, in this case which was one of our initial cases no probe was inserted distally to the anastomosis so we assume that the intima was damaged where the shunt was placed leading to LAD occlusion. Even if anastomosis was patent we feel that this was a technique-related complication and if the patient would not have the second procedure, he would have probably been extubated not having the pneumonia leading to death.

The presented technique is used by a single surgeon in 100% of all the bypass procedures independent of the size of the heart, low ventricular ejection fraction, hypertrophy of left ventricle and size or nature of the coronary vessels.

The aim is to perform the described technique even in demanding procedures, from which the patient would really benefit. However, this is only feasible, when the expertise is gained by always using it.

▌ Summary

With the aim of avoiding cardiopulmonary bypass for coronary artery bypass grafting, off-pump techniques were developed and used in the past. First attempts to standardize the off-pump procedure using a sophisticated device were made in the mid 1990s. The technique was initially used for only grafting of vessels of the anterior wall (LAD, RCA). With increasing experience, several tricks and maneuvers were combined to maintain hemodynamics while tilting the heart to access the coronary vessels of the back wall, thus, enabling complete revascularization, even in extended forms of coronary artery disease. In the present article, a mature technique for OPCAB is presented. To maintain hemodynamics while exposing back wall coronary vessels, pericardial stitches in addition to the Trendelenburg maneuver, right rotation of the operating table, atrial pacing and exposure devices are used. Using a coronary stabilizing device combining pressure and suction and also using coronary shunts, the anastomosis can always be performed in a standard fashion. The mature nature of the presented technique is appreciated by an extremely low conversion rate and an extremely low anastomotic complication rate in the use of this technique on a routine basis.

References

1. Benetti FJ, Ballester C, Sani G, Boonstra P, Grandjean J (1995) Video assisted coronary bypass surgery. J Card Surg 10:620–625
2. Borst C, Jansen EW, Tulleken CA, Gruendemann PF, Mansvelt Beck HJ, van Dongen JW, Hodde KC, Bredee JJ (1996) Coronary artery bypass grafting without cardiopulmonary bypass and without interruption of native coronary flow using a novel anastomosis site restraining device ("Octopus"). J Am Coll Cardiol 27:1356–1364
3. Calafiore AM, Gianmarco GD, Teodori G, Bosco G, D'Annunzio E, Barsotti A, Maddestra N, Paloscia L, Vitolla G, Sciarra A, Fino C, Contini M (1996) Left anterior descending coronary artery grafting via left anterior small thoracotomy without cardiopulmonary bypass. Ann Thorac Surg 61:1658–1665
4. Gulielmos V, Kappert U, Eller M, Sahre H, Alexiou K, Georgi C, Nicolai J, Hartmann N (2003) Improving hemodynamics during off-pump bypass surgery by atrial pacing. The Heart Surgery Forum (in press)
5. Jansen E, Gruendemann P, Borst C et al (1997) Less invasive off-pump CABG using a suction device for immobilization: the 'Octopus' method. Eur J Cardiothorac Surg 12:406–412

6. Kolessov VI (1967) Mammary artery-coronary artery anastomosis as a method of treatment for angina pectoris. J Thorac Cardiovasc Surg 54:535
7. Nicolai J (2003) Anesthetic management. In: Gulielmos V (ed) Beating Heart Bypass Surgery and Minimally Invasive Conduit Harvesting. Cardiosurgical Techniques, Anesthesia Management. Steinkopff, Darmstadt, pp 83–92
8. Reichenspurner H, Gulielmos V, Wunderlich J, Dangel M, Wagner FM, Karbalai P, Schröder C, Pompili M, Stevens J, Schüler S (1997) Port-access coronary artery surgery with the use of cardiopulmonary bypass and cardioplegic arrest – clinical experience with 42 cases. Ann Thorac Surg 65:413–419
9. Stevens JH, Burdon TA, Peters WS, Siegel LC, Pompili MF, Vierra MA, St. Goar FG, Ribakove GH, Mitchell RS, Reitz BA (1996) Port-access coronary artery bypass grafting: a proposed surgical method. J Thorac Cardiovasc Surg 111:567–573

OPCAB for multiple arterial revascularization

J. F. Gummert, J.-F. Légaré, F. W. Mohr

Introduction

The superiority of off-pump coronary artery bypass (OPCAB) versus on-pump coronary revascularization remains to be conclusively proven with only a few randomized studies performed with small groups of patients [1, 15, 18, 19]. However, a significant body of evidence, from large risk-adjusted retrospective studies, has suggested that coronary surgery performed without cardiopulmonary bypass (CPB) may reduce early mortality and major morbidity, such as, neurocognitive dysfunction, stroke, renal insufficiency and are the focus of previous chapters [10, 14]. The present chapter will focus on complete arterial grafting in the setting of OPCAB.

The following topics will be discussed in this chapter: a) the value of arterial grafts in the OPCAB setting, b) perioperative strategies and technical aspects, and c) potential pitfalls of exclusive arterial grafting.

Arterial grafts – the conduits of choice

Most surgeons, when asked, generally accept the value of complete arterial grafting. In fact there are numerous publications that have suggested benefit of arterial grafting particularly with regard to long-term graft patency [7]. Graft occlusion can result in return of disabling angina, the need for re-hospitalization, re-intervention or death [3]. It is well established that patency rates for left internal thoracic artery (left ITA) grafts to the left anterior descending artery (LAD) are excellent compared to saphenous vein grafts (SVG) with patency rates at 10 years of 90% [3]. The short-term graft patency could potentially also be affected by the type of revascularization, since OPCAB surgery appears to be associated with a hypercoagulable state following surgery, thus suggesting that the use of saphenous vein grafts may be more susceptible to thrombosis as compared to arterial grafts [12].

Utilization of ITA grafts has been demonstrated to confer a survival benefit to CABG patients leading to the hypothesis that exclusive arterial revascularization without SVGs would result in improved long-term results following CABG [5]. In support of this, there are numerous published series of patients undergoing CABG with complete arterial revascularization using a variety of arterial conduits (e.g. radial artery, left ITA, right ITA, gastroepiploic) demonstrating feasibility and safety [16]). LYTLE et al. in a large retrospective review of 10 124 patients comparing risk-adjusted outcomes of patients who received 2 ITA grafts with patients receiving only one ITA graft determined that single ITA grafting was an independent predictor of death and re-intervention [13]. Recently a case-matched study comparing the saphenous vein graft (n = 956) to the radial artery graft (n = 478) showed an improved freedom from re-intervention up to 36 months in radial artery conduit patients [6].

The risk factors of embolic complications from an atherosclerotic aorta have been well described and have been shown to correlate with peri-operative neurological complications [9]. The mechanisms by which atherosclerotic material can detach from the aorta and reach the brain include any manipulation of the aorta such as aortic cross clamping, partial occlusion, cannulation, and internal disruption caused by the high velocity jet of blood exiting the aortic cannula. Therefore minimizing any aortic manipulation by avoiding CPB in OPCAB procedures, and more specifically exclusive arterial revascularization using composite grafts by creating a Y or T graft from a pedicled ITA (no touch technique) have therefore been proposed to reduce neurological complications associated with coronary operations [11].

Minor reasons favoring the use of arterial conduits also include versatility (T graft, Y graft, U graft or to aorta), easier to judge length, quality often better than vein, and reduced morbidity of harvesting as compared to lower extremity harvesting [4, 17].

Taken together with the increased potential for improved graft patency, improved survival and fewer neurological complications suggest that complete arterial grafting in selected patients may be superior to conventional revascularization with SVGs.

Perioperative strategies and technical aspects

This technical section will focus on important issues regarding OPCAB complete arterial grafting based on our personal experience and preferred approach. In our center OPCAB procedures are performed routinely by most surgeons. In 2002 out of 1845 isolated coronary patients 569 (=31%) were performed without using the heart-lung machine.

Our choice of conduits is individualized for every patient based on co-morbid factors such as diabetes, peripheral vascular disease, obesity and COPD. Internal thoracic arteries are routinely skeletonized in an effort to avoid sternal wound infections [8] and routinely gently injected with a vasodilator solution of papaverine (intravascular). A radial artery or gastroepiploic artery is harvested as needed using standard described techniques focusing on minimal manipulation of the arterial conduits during harvesting [2]. All radial artery conduits are currently harvested with an ultrasonic cautery system (Ethicon, USA Inc).

Our surgical technique is similar to that used for routine OP-CAB surgery. Two retraction sutures are placed in the posterior pericardium for retraction. We use and have used most of the available retractors and stabilizers for target vessel exposure and stabilization. A 4-0 polypropylene, pledgeted suture is then placed around the target vessel proximal to the anastomotic site and is gently tightened with a tourniquet in order to achieve hemostasis. The coronary arteriotomy is performed 30–60 seconds thereafter, if no significant ECG or hemodynamic disturbance has occurred. Intracoronary shunts are used if the target vessel has a subcritical stenosis, if there are signs of hemodynamic or electrocardiographic instability during vessel occlusion, or if coronary blood flow is excessive and obscuring the field of vision. The anastamosis is constructed as a continuous suture technique with 7-0 or 8-0 monofilament.

There is an ongoing debate about the best sequence of grafting in OBCAB surgery. With complete arterial grafting we generally advise performing the proximal T-Graft anastomosis first in order to assess flow through the anastomosis and then provide inflow to the distal anastomosis i. e., in an effort to avoid proximal anastomosis to the aorta. Our preference is then to perform the left ITA to LAD anastomosis unless not critically stenosed or providing substantial collateral flow to several other territories. The sequence from then is generally first to the most severely stenosed, occluded or collateralized vessels. Judging the length of grafts is also made a little easier with OP-CAB surgery and with arterial grafts which are less prone to kinking than vein conduits. Regarding the proximal right coronary artery anastomosis, we routinely use epicardial pacing and/or shunt if ischemia or bradycardia ensues.

▌Potential pitfalls of complete arterial grafting

There are potential limitations of complete arterial grafting. Arterial conduits are generally smaller than veins and have better vasomotor responses which may result in vascular spasm in the context of high catecholamines and reduce coronary blood flow. This phenomenon can be particularly risky when all coronary blood flow is dependent on a single IMA pedicle such as composite T or Y grafts. Therefore, exclusive arterial grafting is often not advocated in patients with acute coronary syndromes requiring emergency revascularization and inotropic support. However, a clear increase in low-output syndrome with arterial grafts has not been consistently reported in the literature, perhaps because these reports represent selected single-center series without clear criteria and general publication bias [16].

The use of bilateral IMA in diabetic patients who are also obese and have chronic obstructive lung disease remains an important combination of risk factors for sternal wound problems [8]. However, we currently squeletonize all IMA conduits based on evidence suggesting better sternal vascular preservation and potential reduction in sternal wound problems. Our experience with squeletonized IMA and sternal wound problems is currently being evaluated for future publication.

Many issues remain unresolved but are the focus of attention of many groups such as ours. Is there an age limit, for example, where the benefit of arterial grafting is outweighed by the increased technical difficulty and operating time necessary? We believe that patients with the highest risk factors for neurological complications, such as age, would benefit most from OPCAB complete arterial grafting without aortic manipulation.

Summary

In summary OPCAB complete arterial grafting appears feasible, safe and potentially applicable to an increasing number of patients as more evidence for its support accumulates. Ultimately the goals of complete arterial revascularization with OPCAB are to reduce the need for re-intervention, reduce the return of angina, eliminate aortic manipulation, increase the event-free survival and ultimately the overall survival of patients.

References

1. Ascione R, Angelini GD (2003) OPCAB surgery: a voyage of discovery back to the future. Eur Heart J 24(2):121–124
2. Barner HB (1999) The continuing evolution of arterial conduits. Ann Thorac Surg 68(3 Suppl):S1–S8
3. Bourassa MG, Fisher LD, Campeau L, Gillespie MJ, McConney M, Lesperance J (1985) Long-term fate of bypass grafts: the Coronary Artery Surgery Study (CASS) and Montreal Heart Institute experiences. Circulation 72(6 Pt 2):V71–V78
4. Calafiore AM, Contini M, Vitolla G et al (2000) Bilateral internal thoracic artery grafting: long-term clinical and angiographic results of in situ versus Y grafts. J Thorac Cardiovasc Surg 120(5): 990–996
5. Cameron A, Davis KB, Green G, Schaff HV (1996) Coronary bypass surgery with internal-thoracic-artery grafts – effects on survival over a 15-year period. N Engl J Med 334(4):216–219
6. Cohen G, Tamariz MG, Sever JY et al (2001) The radial artery versus the saphenous vein graft in contemporary CABG: a case-matched study. Ann Thorac Surg 71(1):180–185
7. Fitzgibbon GM, Kafka HP, Leach AJ, Keon WJ, Hooper GD, Burton JR (1996) Coronary bypass graft fate and patient outcome: angiographic follow-up of 5065 grafts related to survival and reoperation in 1,388 patients during 25 years. J Am Coll Cardiol 28(3): 616–626
8. Gummert JF, Barten MJ, Hans C et al (2002) Mediastinitis and cardiac surgery – an updated risk factor analysis in 10 373 consecutive adult patients. Thorac Cardiovasc Surg 50(2):87–91

9. Hammon JW Jr, Stump DA, Kon ND et al (1997) Risk factors and solutions for the development of neurobehavioral changes after coronary artery bypass grafting. Ann Thorac Surg 63(6):1613–1618

10. Hart JC, Puskas JD, Sabik JF III (2002) Off-pump coronary revascularization: current state of the art. Semin Thorac Cardiovasc Surg 14(1):70–81

11. Kim KB, Kang CH, Chang WI et al (2002) Off-pump coronary artery bypass with complete avoidance of aortic manipulation. Ann Thorac Surg 74(4):S1377–S1382

12. Kim KB, Lim C, Lee C et al (2001) Off-pump coronary artery bypass may decrease the patency of saphenous vein grafts. Ann Thorac Surg 72(3):S1033–S1037

13. Lytle BW, Blackstone EH, Loop FD et al (1999) Two internal thoracic artery grafts are better than one. J Thorac Cardiovasc Surg 117(5):855–872

14. Magee MJ, Jablonski KA, Stamou SC et al (2002) Elimination of cardiopulmonary bypass improves early survival for multivessel coronary artery bypass patients. Ann Thorac Surg 73(4):1196–1202

15. Nathoe HM, van Dijk D, Jansen EW et al (2003) A comparison of on-pump and off-pump coronary bypass surgery in low-risk patients. N Engl J Med 348(5):394–402

16. Tector AJ, McDonald ML, Kress DC, Downey FX, Schmahl TM (2001) Purely internal thoracic artery grafts: outcomes. Ann Thorac Surg 72(2):450–455

17. Tran HM, Paterson HS, Meldrum-Hanna W, Chard RB (1998) Tunnelling versus open harvest technique in obtaining venous conduits for coronary bypass surgery. Eur J Cardiothorac Surg 14(6): 602–606

18. van Dijk D, de Jaegere PP (2002) Neuropsychological outcome after off-pump versus on-pump coronary bypass surgery: the octopus randomized trial. Circulation 105(21):E179

19. van Dijk D, Nierich AP, Jansen EW et al (2001) Early outcome after off-pump versus on-pump coronary bypass surgery: results from a randomized study. Circulation 104(15):1761–1766

CHAPTER 3 MIDCAB

MIDCAB – anesthesia management

B. BEIN, P. H. TONNER

Introduction

The MIDCAB (minimally invasive direct coronary artery by-pass) procedure is an off-pump cardiac surgical approach performing the revascularization of the left anterior descendent coronary artery (LAD) by a left internal mammary artery (IMA) graft on the beating heart [2]. The aim of this type of surgery is to minimize surgical trauma, to avoid the vigorous inflammatory response after cardiopulmonary bypass (CPB) and to realize effective fast tracking.

Surgical technique and posture

Currently, there are mainly two types of surgical technique for the MIDCAB procedure. The first uses thoracoscopic, video-assisted harvesting of the IMA prior to the anastomosis to the LAD via left anterior thoracotomy. For the endoscopic IMA, dissection ports for camera, scalpel and carbon dioxide insufflator are inserted via the T3 to T6 intercostal spaces. For optimizing heart exposure, CO_2 (pressure 12–14 mmHg) is insufflated in the thoracic cavity, thus, increasing the distance between the heart and the thoracic wall [13].

The second approach is performed via a left anterolateral minithoracotomy in the 4th or 5th intercostal space. The dissection and harvesting of the IMA are performed under direct sight via a special rib retractor enabling sufficient exposure of the vessel.

Prior to clamping the LAD, 100 I.E./kg of unfractioned heparin is administered aiming for an activated clotting time (ACT) of approximately 200 seconds to facilitate anastomosis. After reestablishment of blood flow, the heparin is antagonized (usually one half to two thirds of the initial dose), depending on the clinical coagulation problems.

Both techniques require a motionless field to facilitate anastomosis on the beating heart. A variety of stabilizers are available to ensure a fixed heart surface during the vessel suture.

To control back bleeding, the LAD is temporarily closed distally and proximally by silastic sutures. During the entire procedure a collapse of the left lung and one-lung ventilation is necessary to enable surgical access.

Patients are positioned in the lateral tilt position (left thorax 30° elevated). Dependent upon the surgical approach, arms are supported adjacent to the body (minithoracotomy) or free-draped to facilitate instrumentation (endoscopic procedure). One lower limb is exposed for surgical access to enable venous graft harvesting (for lengthening the mammary graft if necessary) and institution of cardiopulmonary bypass in case of an emergency. The anesthesiologist should be aware of unphysiological positioning and ensure that neurological injury is avoided.

▊ Patient selection and preoperative evaluation

Generally there are two very different patient populations who would benefit from the MIDCAB procedure. The first represents patients with an isolated one vessel disease of the LAD. These patients are generally in adequate physical condition with a normal left ventricular ejection fraction (EF) and no significant concomitant disease of other organ systems. The respiratory system is commonly unaffected by obstructive and/or restrictive impairment, which is especially important regarding prolonged one-lung ventilation. Arrhythmias are unusual in this patient population.

The second group is represented by severely impaired patients, who are thought not to be suitable for coronary artery bypass grafting (CABG) with cardiopulmonary bypass. These patients often suffer from multivessel disease with markedly reduced EF and a history of myocardial infarction and congestive heart failure. Multiple organ systems are affected including cerebrovascular, renal and respiratory disease. Atrial fibrillation, implanted pacemakers and cardioverters are frequently found. Hence, the MIDCAB procedure in these patients is to some extent a palliative attempt to optimize cardiac oxygen supply.

Regardless of patient population, preoperative anesthetic evaluation has to comprise thorough physical examination and review of the patient's medical records. In addition to routine technical examinations (electrocardiogram, chest x-ray, laboratory examinations), the coronary angiography report with specification of the type and extent of the affected vessels as well as a characterization of left ventricular performance must be available to the anesthesiologist. In the case of overt respiratory impairment arterial blood gas analysis and pulmonary function tests (including forced vital capacity FVC and forced one second capacity FEV1) are necessary to stratify the individual patient's risk. Though the value of pulmonary function testing remains controversial with regard to postoperative ventilatory failure and outcome [5], the rationale in the MIDCAB population is to identify patients in which there is the potential for optimizing airflow obstruction preoperatively and patients who will most probably not tolerate prolonged one-lung ventilation of the extent required for this type of surgery.

Since insertion of a double lumen tube is preferable for one-lung ventilation, special care has to be taken of documented difficult intubations and clinical signs of possible intubation difficulties (i.e., Mallampati classification). The use of an Univent^{TM} tube should be considered if intubation difficulties are assumed.

Serum electrolytes, especially potassium should be in the normal range preoperatively. To account for possible, deleterious arrhythmic episodes during surgery external defibrillator pads may be attached to the chest wall.

Perioperative medications should be checked for timely discontinuation of antiplatelet agents (at least 5 days prior to surgery). In contrast, β-blockade should be continued or initiated perioperatively. Alternatively, a_2-adrenoceptor agonists can be used for premedication in conjunction with benzodiazepines (i.e., 2 µg/kg clonidine and 0.1 mg/kg midazolam).

It has been shown that patients who have undergone coronary angioplasty within 2 weeks prior to non-cardiac surgery are exposed to an increased risk of perioperative myocardial events and death. Despite lacking data for patients scheduled for cardiac surgery, the period between angioplasty and the MIDCAB procedure may be of paramount importance [9].

▌ Anesthetic management and monitoring

The scope of anesthetic management for the MIDCAB procedure comprises several areas of concern: hemodynamic stability particularly during anastomosis of LAD and IMA; adequate tissue oxygenation during one-lung ventilation; prevention of myocardial ischemia; adequate postoperative analgesia and temperature homeostasis.

Hemodynamic stability is crucial to avoid insufficient coronary artery perfusion pressure during LAD clamping, when the myocardium is at risk for ischemia and when blood supply to the lateral wall is sustained by collaterals of the circumflex or right coronary artery. Several devices for continuous cardiac output (CCO) measurement are available, the pulmonary artery catheter being the most invasive device. Pulse contour analysis (PiCCO^{TM}, Pulsion, Munich, Germany) appears to be a reliable alternative [6]. Cardiac output monitoring should be adapted to the individual patient's needs. While a patient in a fairly good condition can be managed without CCO measurement, a patient scheduled for a palliative MIDCAB procedure will require CCO monitoring in combination with transesophageal echocardiography for visualization of regional mall motion abnormalities and assessment of left ventricular function.

Although one-lung ventilation is not essential for the MIDCAB surgical approach, it is used in our institution to facilitate surgery. Independent of the individual patient's physical condition (i.e., chronic obstructive lung disease and asthma), single lung ventilation (SLV) may cause significant oliguria, a reduction in cardiac output, may increase pulmonary artery pressure and pulmonary artery resistance [1]. Furthermore, prolonged one-lung ventilation can result in pulmonal fluid sequestration and edema, and a marked ventilation-perfusion mismatch. Severely bronchospastic patients may not tolerate one-lung ventilation.

To minimize changes associated with SLV, several precautions should be accomplished. During SLV the fraction of inspired oxygen (FiO_2) is adjusted to 1.0. Apneic oxygenation (2 l/min O_2) together with continuous positive airway pressure (CPAP, 5 cm H_2O) is applied to the collapsed lung via a special oxygenation device (Broncho-Cath^{TM} CPAP system, Mallinckrodt Medical, Athlone, Ireland) [15]. Despite these efforts, intermittent ventilation of the collapsed lung may be inevitable in some patients.

Generally a pressure-controlled ventilation mode with a peak airway pressure below 30 cm H_2O together with an extended time interval for expiration (i.e., I:E ratio 1:3) is best suitable for SLV [15].

Prevention of myocardial ischemia is an issue of paramount importance in MIDCAB. If the LAD is not totally occluded, disruption of blood flow during anastomosis will render the tissue perfused by this coronary artery susceptible for ischemia and hypoxia. Five lead ECG with automatic ST segment trend analysis is helpful for detecting acute changes, but may be confused by improper placement of the lateral chest lead (i.e., V5) due to the extension of the surgical field. Transesophageal echocardiography is superior, as wall motion abnormalities are more sensitive for myocardial ischemia than the ECG. TEE findings however may be hampered by stabilizers used for the motionless surgical field, thus, precluding assessment of the myocardial contractility in this area [11].

Currently there are two major attempts to protect the myocardium against ischemia: ischemic preconditioning and the administration of volatile anesthetics. Ischemic preconditioning is performed by clamping the LAD for a short period (i.e., 2 minutes) followed by a reperfusion phase (i.e., 3 minutes) prior to the definite clamping during the anastomosis [7].

Volatile anesthetics (i.e., 1 MAC, sevoflurane) exert their cardioprotective effect through the K^+-dependent ATP channels [14]. Recently evolving evidence suggests that volatile anesthetics may be beneficial in cardiac surgery compared to intravenous anesthesia [3].

If hemodynamic instability and/or signs of severe myocardial ischemia persist despite these efforts, shunt insertion is an alternative.

Generally, anesthesia should be maintained with short acting drugs to enable fast tracking. At our institution we use a combination of sevoflurane (1 MAC) in an air/oxygen mixture and remifentanil (0.2 to 0.5 µg/kg/min). Other regimens including propofol and sufentanil have been advocated for MIDCAB as well. Effective pain control is another important issue in preventing myocardial ischemia. The sympathetic response provoked by postoperative pain may result in the release of catecholamines and other stress hormones. Lateral thoracotomy is apparently more painful than median sternotomy [4]. Various approaches to optimal pain control are described in the literature including thoracic epidural anesthesia (TEA), intercostal blockade and intrapleural catheter placement [8]. Currently there are no data demonstrating an clear advantage of one method over the others. At our institution we apply a multimodal concept including NSAID (1 g paracetamol rectally during induction of anaesthesia, 1 g novaminsulfone prior to emergence from anesthesia) and intercostal blockades covering the segments T4–T6 (37.5 mg ropivacain per segment) upon wound closure. Additionally, a_2-adrenozeptor-agonists (i.e., 150 µg clonidine) are administered to prevent tachycardia and hypertension [12].

Accidental hypothermia has been shown to exert various adverse effects perioperatively. Shivering can increase oxygen consumption dramatically, while hypothermia may impede fast tracking [10]. We use a special ambient air warmer which is positioned adjacent to the patient's lateral body surface (Bair Hugger 560 Cath Lab™, Augustine Medical, Minnesota, USA). All intravenous fluids are warmed and the temperature of the operating theater is raised to 24 °C.

Conclusion

The MIDCAB procedure has evolved from a novel off-pump cardiac surgical approach to an established procedure. Anesthetic considerations should address the special issues of this type of surgery. Prolonged single lung ventilation, risk of myocardial ischemia and limited access to the heart in the case of arrhythmias or severe bleeding are the most important points. Anesthesia management should facilitate fast tracking by an adequate choice of short acting drugs. To fully realize the benefits of the pharmacologic advances, an individually tailored concept for postoperative pain control has to be established. a_2-adrenoreptor-agonists (i.e., clonidine) may be beneficial for attenuation of intraoperative sympathetic stress response and as a basis for effective postoperative pain control.

References

1. Boldt J, Papsdorf M, Uphus D, Muller M, Hempelmann G (1997) Changes in regulators of the circulation in patients undergoing lung surgery. Br J Anaesth 79:733–739
2. Cremer J, Wittwer T, Boning A, Anssar M, Kofidis T, Zuk J, Mehler D, Haverich A (1999) [Minimally invasive revascularization of the anterior myocardial vessels on a beating heart]. Z Kardiol 88 (Suppl 4):S2–S9
3. De Hert SG, ten Broecke PW, Mertens E, Van Sommeren EW, De Blier IG, Stockman BA, Rodrigus IE (2002) Sevoflurane but not propofol preserves myocardial function in coronary surgery patients. Anesthesiology 97:42–49
4. Diegeler A, Walther T, Metz S, Falk V, Krakor R, Autschbach R, Mohr FW (1999) Comparison of MIDCAP versus conventional CABG surgery regarding pain and quality of life. Heart Surg Forum 2:290–295
5. Gass GD, Olsen GN (1986) Preoperative pulmonary function testing to predict postoperative morbidity and mortality. Chest 89:127–135
6. Goedje O, Hoeke K, Lichtwarck-Aschoff M, Faltchauser A, Lamm P, Reichart B (1999) Continuous cardiac output by femoral arterial thermodilution calibrated pulse contour analysis: comparison with pulmonary arterial thermodilution. Crit Care Med, 27: 2407–2412.
7. Hawaleshka A, Jacobsohn E (1998) Ischaemic preconditioning: mechanisms and potential clinical applications. Can J Anaesth 45:670–682
8. Heres EK, Marquez J, Malkowski MJ, Magovern JA, Gravlee GP (1998) Minimally invasive direct coronary artery bypass: anesthetic, monitoring, and pain control considerations. J Cardiothorac Vasc Anesth 12:385–389
9. Kaluza GL, Joseph J, Lee JR, Raizner ME, Raizner AE (2000) Catastrophic outcomes of noncardiac surgery soon after coronary stenting. J Am Coll Cardiol 35:1288–1294
10. Leslie K, Sessler DI (1998) The implications of hypothermia for early tracheal extubation following cardiac surgery. J Cardiothorac Vasc Anesth 12:30–34; discussion 41–34
11. Mehta Y, Juneja R, Dhole S (1999) Transesophageal echocardiography in MIDCAB: pitfalls. J Cardiothorac Vasc Anesth 13:115–116

12. Scholz J, Tonner PH (1996) [Alpha 2-adrenoreceptor agonists – horse or donkey?]. Anasthesiol Intensivmed Notfallmed Schmerzther 31:401–403
13. Subramanian VA, McCabe JC, Geller CM (1997) Minimally invasive direct coronary artery bypass grafting: two-year clinical experience. Ann Thorac Surg 64:1648–1653; discussion 1654–1645
14. Zaugg M, Lucchinetti E, Spahn DR, Pasch T, Schaub MC (2002) Volatile anesthetics mimic cardiac preconditioning by priming the activation of mitochondrial K(ATP) channels via multiple signaling pathways. Anesthesiology 97:4–14
15. Zollinger A (1999) [Anesthesia in thoracic surgery]. Anaesthesist 48:193–204

MIDCAB – small access bypass surgery

J. Cremer, S. Fraund

Introduction

After its first introduction in 1967 by Kolesov, MIDCAB regained new interest in the early 1990s. At that time Benetti, Calafiore, Subramanian and Boonstra [1–3, 13] reported on LIMA grafting to the LAD through a similar minithoracotomy using specialized equipment for intrathoracic exposure and local immobilization of the target area. Along with the availability of suitable equipment a broad interest for MIDCAB grafting developed, as MIDCAB combines the two major procedural advantages of beating off-pump surgery and minimal access. Beside the 'original' MIDCAB procedure (beating heart off-pump, anterior minithoracotomy, LIMA-LAD bypass) several modifications have been attempted including parasternal incisions and inferior ministernotomies [7, 9, 12]. Sometimes mobilization or partial resection of one or two ribs became necessary.

The following standardization of the procedure allows for adequate and reproducible results in experienced hands (Table 1).

Surgical access and IMA preparation

The patient is positioned in a 30-degree supine position with elevation of the left hemithorax and draped for immediate conversion to conventional procedure enabling sternotomy, saphe-

Table 1. Sequences of the surgical steps of the MIDCAB procedure

- Skin incision
- Single-lung ventilation
- Preparation of the anterior pleural attachment
- LIMA preparation
- Mobilization of the pre-pericardial fat
- L-shaped pericardial incision
- LAD identification
- Estimation of required LIMA length
- Dissection of the distal LIMA
- Stay sutures for the LIMA pedicle
- Distal LIMA preparation and flow check
- Pericardial traction sutures
- Optimization of LAD exposure
- Placement of the stabilizer
- LAD preparation
- Placement of tourniquet sutures
- Test occlusion of the LAD
- LAD incision
- Performance of the anastomoses
- Check of the anastomoses
- Removal of the tourniquets
- Fixation sutures for the distal pedicle
- Removal of the stabilizer
- Check for LIMA course
- Refixation of the pre-pericardial fat to the mediastinum
- Placement of a pleural drainage tube
- Double lung ventilation
- Wound closure

nous vein harvest and exposure of the femoral vessels. Ventilation is prepared for single right lung ventilation using double lumen tubes or blocker catheters.

Depending on the projection of the heart's silhouette in relation to the thorax and the coronary anatomy (distal anastomoses) on the chest x-ray the 4th or 5th interspace is selected for incision. In females the skin becomes incised in the submammary fold and in males there should be a distance of at least 2 centimeters between the incision and the nipple (Fig. 1). Initially a horizontally spreading suitable retractor is introduced. Before starting with the preparation of the LIMA pedicle the anterior attachments of the mediastinum to the anterior chest wall close to the IMA course are dissected. Thereafter the endothoracic fascia becomes transsected under the next upper rib at a safe distance to the IMA facilitating identification of the correct plane of tissue. As it is significantly more difficult

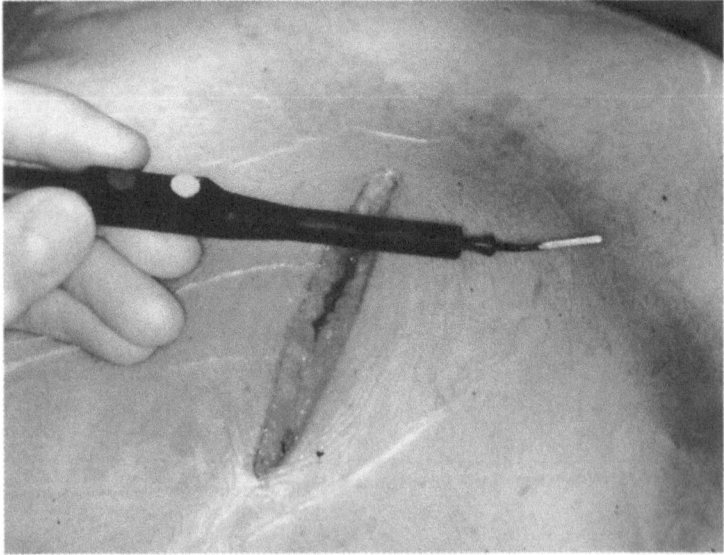

Fig. 1. Submammary skin incision entering the 4th or 5th interspace

to prepare the IMA from lateral the preparation in this layer is continued medially beyond the IMA vessels and distally before transsecting the medial part of the fascia. Then the retractor has to be switched to a vertically opening system (e.g., Thora-LIFT, Vascular Therapies, Norwalk, CT).

Under direct vision the preparation is extended usually to get a total pedicle length of 12–14 cm allowing for a tension-free bypass course. It does not appear necessary to have complete proximal preparation and dissect all side branches. With systemic heparinization (100 IU/kg body weight) and external application of papaverin, the left IMA remains perfused until the LAD anastomotic site is defined.

Changing back again to a horizontal spreader the pre-pericardial fat tissue is mobilized and remains laterally attached to the pericardium. Different from earlier techniques the pre-pericardial fat tissue is no longer excised. Then the pericardium becomes incised using a rectangular fashion followed by exploration of the heart surface with evaluation of the condition and

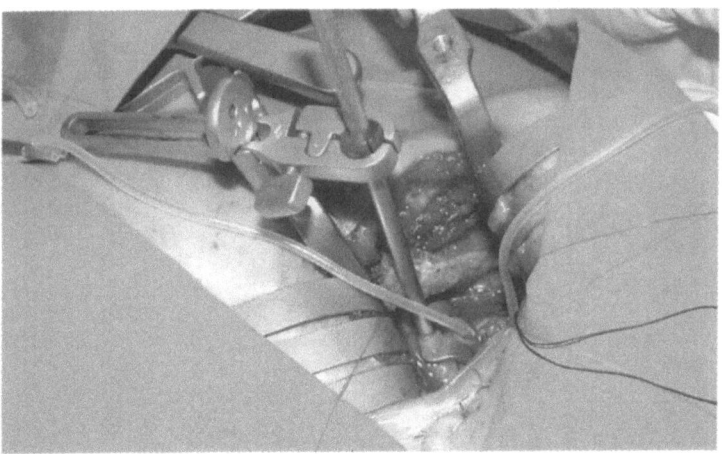

Fig. 2. LIMA distally incised for anastomosis, mechanical stabilizer in position, tourniquet sutures occluded

course of the LAD. To avoid mal-connection, verification of the septal area by palpation alone is mandatory. In case the pedicle length corresponds with the intended anastomotic region, the left IMA is dissected and distally prepared for anastomosing. Thereby the distal pedicle is presented with the aid of two stay sutures (5/0 prolene) at the medial angle of the incision and the vessel is clamped with an a-traumatic microvascular bulldog clamp arranged with a transthoracic suture. Using two or three pledgeted pericardial traction sutures the heart is rotated to present the LAD favorably in the mid of the surgical field. Applying a mechanical stabilizer the LAD is prepared and encircled by two 4/0 polypropylene sutures combined with a very flexible silicon tube for gentle snaring (Fig. 2). After proximal occlusion for

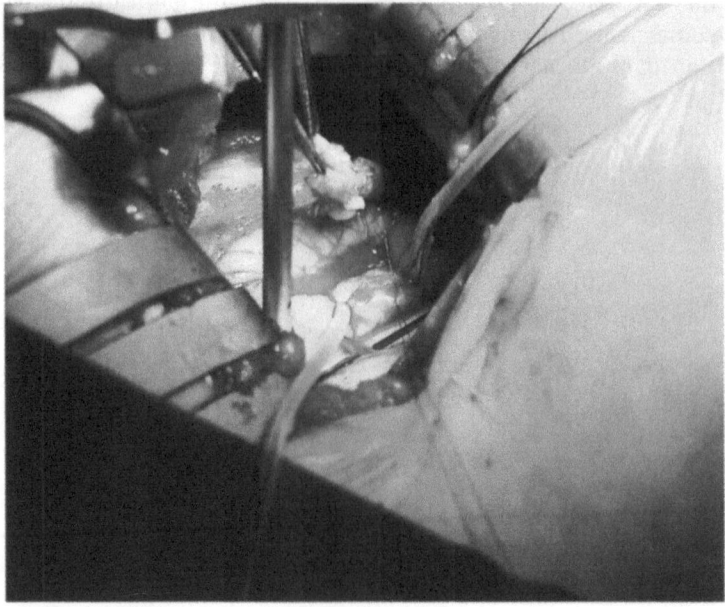

Fig. 3. Anastomosis: after the first 5 stitches the LIMA is approximated for completion of the sutureline

two minutes the LAD becomes incised and depending on collateral flow the distal tourniquet is gently adjusted. Additional visualization of vascular structures is achieved with a blowing device. The anastomosis is created with only one continuous 8/0 polypropylene suture (75 cm) starting two contralateral stitches before the heel. Going around the heel, five stitches are symmetrically placed (Fig. 3). Then the left IMA is approximated to the LAD and the anastomosis becomes completed from the contra lateral site. Thereafter the distal tourniquet is released first to enable de-airing through side branches (Fig. 4). Under conversion of the anticoagulation the anastomosis and the IMA pedicle is checked for bleeding and adequate course. The distal pedicle part becomes fixed to the epicardium with several 5/0 stitches (fascia up). If there is no bleeding the pre-pericardial fat tissue, which has been mobilized, is re-fixated to the mediastinum with several stitches. Thus, the anastomosis and the distal IMA are covered by

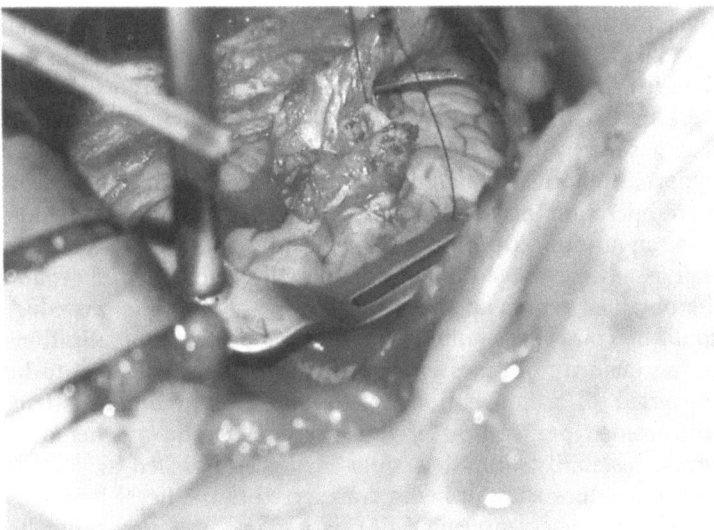

Fig. 4. Completed LIMA-LAD bypass, stabilizer still in position, tourniquet sutures loosened

tissue and potential adhesion of the anastomosed region to the anterior thoracic wall is prevented. One angled thoracic draining tube is placed and the pre-thoracic tissue is closed with single stitches. Especially in situations with limited intra-thoracic space it may be advantageous to insert the drainage tube right after performance of the minithoracotomy. Re-adapting the muscle, the subcutaneous tissue and the skin secondary herniation of the lung should be effectively prevented. Pericostal sutures are not necessary. For perioperative pain reduction intercostal blockade or pleural anaesthetic treatment may be suitable. Most of our patients are extubated at the end of the procedure and transferred spontaneously breathing to the intensive care unit for at least several hours [8].

Clinical results

Over the last four years 320 patients (231 male/89 female, mean age 62.3 ± 10.3 years) have undergone MIDCAB grafting in our department under various conditions. The majority of patients were in a stable clinical situation (Table 2), but several patients had a severely depressed left ventricular function, pulmonary hypertension, unstable angina, acute coronary syndrome, cardiac re-operation, or were on preoperative IABP-support. In addition, significant co-morbidities were present in many cases as well as advanced age (Table 3). Especially with this background the obtained results appear absolutely satisfying. The procedure could be completed without major intraoperative complications in the majority of cases except for one patient, who had to be converted to a conventional procedure and another patient, who needed preparation of the groin vessels due to hemodynamic instability, but who could finally be finished as a MIBCAB procedure without being transferred to the heart-lung machine. However, ventricular fibrillation in two cases could be successfully converted into regular rhythm allowing for continuation of the MIDCAB procedure. Perioperative myocardial

Table 2. Cardiac findings of the 320 MIDCAB patients

Parameters	N 320 (%)
One-vessel disease	191 (59.7)
Two-vessel disease*	94 (29.3)
Three-vessel disease*	35 (11)
LV-EF < 30%	19 (6.0)
Unstable Angina	36 (11.3)
Previous cardiac surgery	24 (7.5)
Previous PTCA/Stenting of LAD	68 (21.3)
Previous myocardial infarction	127 (40)
Preoperative IABP	1 (0.3)
Atrial fibrillation	19 (6)
Pulmonary hypertension	11 (3.4)

* The high percentage of 2- and 3-vessel disease is explained by a collective comprising patients with 2- or 3-vessel disease due to preoperatively performed PTCA/stent grafting of a vessel other than the LAD, of patients who had coronary artery bypass grafting before with now a predominantly closed LAD graft, of patients planned for postoperative hybrid procedures, patients with scar tissue in other areas and in one special case MIDCAB was performed as the final option in an 81-year old patient suffering from acute anterior wall infarction. Therefore, these patients are predominantly suffering from functional one-vessel disease. *LV-EF* left ventricular ejection fraction; *PTCA* percutaneous coronary angioplasty; *LAD* left anterior descending; *IABP* intraaortic balloon pump

infarction occurred in two (0.6%) patients. Re-exploration for bleeding became necessary 6 (1.8%) times. Prolonged ventilation beyond 2 days was necessary in 6 patients. Four patients died in the hospital during their early postoperative stay. Reasons were cardiac failure in 1 patient (87 years, preoperative IABP due to acute myocardial infarction), respiratory failure with consecutive sepsis in another patient and sudden death in two patients.

Table 3. Significant preoperative non-cardiac organ dysfunction and comorbidities of the 320 patients

Comorbidities	N 320 (%)
Organ dysfunction	
▮ COPD	18 (5.6)
▮ Renal insufficiency	15 (4.7)
▮ Diabetes	52 (16.3)
▮ BMI ≥30	60 (18.8)
Vascular disease	
▮ Carotid artery stenosis	16 (5.0)
▮ Arterial vascular disease	27 (8.4)
▮ Intracranial artery stenosis	6 (1.9)
Neurological disorders	
▮ Stroke	4 (1.3)
Organ dysfunction	
▮ Malignancies	7 (2.2)

COPD chronic obstructive pulmonary disease; BMI body mass index

Postoperative wound infections were restricted to obese patients. Preferentially females with largely developed breasts (20 of 89 female patients had a BMI ≥30 kg/m^2) had a significant incidence of wound complications (2.8%), one male patient developed an intercostal hernia. Since modification of the anesthesiological management aiming at fast track recovery, the majority of patients (82.5%) could be extubated on the table at the end of the operation allowing regularly for an early transfer to the regular ward within hours.

■ Discussion

■ Surgical access

Under various options to open the chest for a MIDCAB procedure, the minithoracotomy combines several advantages. First, there is no damage of bony structures for most cases and the thoracic stability is absolutely preserved. In addition, there is good access to both the IMA and the LAD. In case of impaired exposition the incision can be expanded. In comparison medial ministernotomies have some degree of bone damage and have limitations in presenting the lateral LAD. Parasternal incisions as earlier used by some groups require transsection or even partial resection of cartilaginous parts of the ribs. However, it has to be admitted that minithoracotomies may be more painful for some time compared to median or para-median incisions [11, 14].

■ LIMA harvest

With some training it is almost always possible to harvest the IMA entering the chest through an anterior minithoracotomy. Using conventional surgical instruments, we favor the LIMA preparation by use of a specially designed commercially available eletrocautery handgrip with different extensions and a very small malleable tip. Especially in female patients with a small chest or in obese patients it may be necessary to have some upward traction on the retractor with the help of the assistant. Sometimes initial removal of the median pre-pericardial fat gives significantly more space and makes access to the IMA easier. Additional supportive techniques, like intrathoracic illumination and continuous intrathoracic suction, are not necessary nor are videoscopic control and instrumentation. Gentle handling of the IMA appears to be even more important than in conventional surgery.

▌ LAD exposure

Especially in combination with an anterior minithoracotomy the LAD can be located in the mid of the surgical field by use of 2 or 3 pledgeted pericardial traction sutures. Stabilization can be obtained by pressure or suction devices. Even with significant pressure to the anterior myocardial wall, hemodynamics should remain sufficiently stable. In contrast to other groups we still rely on tourniquet sutures for LAD occlusion to obtain a bloodless field. However, we usually start with a proximal test occlusion of two minutes and open the LAD directly thereafter. Depending on the distal back flow, the distal tourniquet is gently adjusted. From to the experience of our group the use of shunts or intravascular occluders is usually not required but shunts should be immediately available in case of ventricular arrhythmias and progressive ECG deterioration. Otherwise we prefer to avoid any intravascular manipulation. Additional persistant bleeding is controlled by blowing devices. Even with up to about 20 minutes or more of LAD occlusion a relevant anterior ischemia does not occur. This is probably due to collateral flow and the much more distal LAD occlusion when compared to interventional LAD treatment by PTCA.

▌ Anastomosis and pedicle course

Even though several specific suture techniques, like double suture parachute techniques have been described we prefer a conventional no touch technique with only one 8/0 polypropylene suture to fulfill the same quality standards for anastomosing techniques, like in conventional surgery. In comparison to conventional coronary surgery using sternotomies the mediastinum remains anterior connected to the chest wall resulting in a relatively more anterior position of the anastomosis and the IMA. As assessed by control angiographies this may be responsible for a secondary re-fixation of the distal IMA pedicle to the chest wall potentially resulting in shear stress and tension for the anastomosis. We therefore recently changed our technique and started mediastinal re-fixation of the initially laterally mobilized pre-pericardial fat above the anastomosis and the distal IMA to adequately protect of these structures.

Comment

Even though the numbers of annually performed MIDCAB procedures in Germany decreased steadily over the last few years the surgical technique appears to be standardized and adequately safe with good success for the patient [4–6, 10]. It still represents a surgically demanding procedure which belongs just in experienced hands. As a routine approach in adequately large numbers it represents an extremely cost effective procedure, especially under the reimbursement conditions of the upcoming DRG system.

References

1. Benetti FJ, Naselli G, Wood M, Geffner L (1991) Direct myocardial revascularization without extracorporeal circulation. Experience in 700 patients. Chest 100:312–316
2. Boonstra PW, Grandjean JG, Mariani MA (1997) Improved method for direct coronary grafting without CPB via anterolateral small thoracotomy. Ann Thorac Surg 63(2):567–569
3. Calafiori AM, Di Gammarco G, Teodori G et al. (1996) Left anterior descending coronary artery grafting via left anterior small thoracotomy without cardiopulmonary bypass. Ann Thorac Surg 61: 1658–1665
4. Cremer J, Mügge A, Wittwer T, Böning A, Kim P, Kofides T, Drexler H, Haverich A (1999) Early angiographic results after revascularization by minimally invasive direct coronary artery bypass (MIDCAB). Eur J Cardiothorac Surg Apr 15(4):383–387

5. Diegeler A, Matin M, Falk V, Binner C, Walther T, Autschbach R Mohr FW (1999) Quality assessment in minimally invasive coronary artery bypass grafting. Eur J Cardiothorac Surg Nov 16 (Suppl 2):S67–S72

6. Diegeler A, Walther T, Metz S, Falk V, Krakor R, Autschbach R, Mohr FW (1999) Comparison of MIDCAB versus conventional CABG surgery regarding pain and quality of life. Heart Surg Forum 2(4):290–295

7. Dullum MK, Block J, Qazi A, Shawl F, Benetti F (1999) Xiphoid MIDCAB: report of technique and experience with a less invasive MIDCAB procedure. Heart Surg Forum 2(1):77–81

8. Fraund S, Behnke H, Böning A, Cremer C (2002) Immediate postoperative extubation after minimally invasive direct coronary artery surgery (MIDCAB). Interactive Cardiovasc and Thorac Surg 1:41–45

9. Grandjean JG, Canosa C, Mariani MA, Boonstra PW (1999) Reversed – J inferior sternotomy for beating heart coronary surgery. Ann Thorac Surg May 67(5):1505–1506

10. Mack MJ, Magovern JA, Acuff TA, Landreneau RJ, Tennison DM, Tinnermann EJ, Osborne JA (1999) Results of graft patency by immediate angiography in minimally invasive coronary artery surgery. Ann Thorac Surg Aug 68(2):383–389

11. Ng PC, Chua AN, Swanson MS, Koutlas TC, Chitwood WR Jr, Elbeery JR (2000) Anterior thoracotomy wound complications in minimally invasive direct coronary artery bypass. Ann Thorac Surg May 69(5):1338–1340

12. Riess FC, Bleese N, Riess AG (1999) A new method for coronary occlusion and local stabilization during minimally invasive LIMA-to-LAD bypass. Eur J Cardiothorac Surg 15(2):206–208

13. Subramanian VA, McCabe JC, Geller CM (1997) Minimally invasive direct coronary artery bypass grafting: two year clinical experience. Ann Thorac Surg 64:1648–653

14. Trehan N, Malhotra R, Mishra Y, Shrivastva S, Kohli V, Mehta Y (2000) Comparison of ministernotomy with minithoracotomy regarding postoperative pain and internal mammary artery characteristics. Heart Surg Forum 3(4):300–306

Minimal invasive direct coronary artery bypass grafting via partial inferior sternotomy

K. HAKIM, J. BÖRGERMANN

Introduction

Today, treatment of single vessel coronary artery disease is primarily the realm of catheter intervention. A number of current studies compared revascularization of the left anterior descending (LAD) coronary artery by percutaneous transluminal coronary angioplasty (PTCA, with or without stent placement) with coronary artery bypass grafting (CABG) using the internal thoracic artery (ITA). The PTCA groups showed higher reintervention rates and in some studies an increased incidence of postinterventional myocardial infarctions [8–10]. Despite these observations and although the long-term results of ITA grafts are excellent [13, 14], most patients will favor the less invasive approach when given the choice between PTCA and CABG. Yet surgical revascularization of the LAD with an ITA graft can also be accomplished via a minimal invasive approach without extracorporeal circulation (ECC), using a technique called minimal invasive direct coronary artery bypass grafting (MIDCAB). This technique could fill a gap in the treatment options and may at the same time allow surgical myocardial revascularization in high-risk patients. Initial data of a current randomized study show that on 6-month follow-up, revascularization by MIDCAB compares favorably with catheter interventional stent implantation when freedom of angina pectoris (79 vs. 62%) and reintervention rates (8 vs. 29%) are used as endpoints [7].

In 1967, Vassili Kolessov first described minimal invasive revascularization of the LAD with the left internal thoracic artery (LITA), using a beating heart technique and a left anterior thoracotomy for exposure [12]. This method was further developed in the mid-1990s when minimal invasive cardiac surgery began to gain popularity. A number of authors describe the surgical strategies and results achieved with the left anterior small thoracotomy (LAST) approach to MIDCAB revascularization of the LAD [1, 4, 5, 16, 17]. For reasons of surgical exposure, the MIDCAB technique is only feasible for patients with single vessel coronary artery disease limited to the LAD. In addition, the method is associated with a number of other limitations and disadvantages [6], one of which is the aggravated pain after lateral thoracotomies compared to (partial) sternotomies [18].

Surgical access via ministernotomy or partial sternotomy has been described as a minimal invasive approach to heart surgery with or without ECC [2, 15, 19]. A number of modifications of the ministernotomy approach permit exposure of the aortic valve (upper T mini-sternotomy) [11] or the coronary arteries (partial inferior sternotomy) [3]. In our experience, the main advantages of partial inferior sternotomy versus other types of minimal invasive access techniques for coronary artery surgery include:

▌ Good exposure of the mid and distal LAD and diagonal branches,

▌ access to the right coronary artery (RCA) through the same approach,

▌ LITA and/or RITA can be dissected under direct vision for their entire course while pleural integrity is preserved,

▌ no need for single lung ventilation,

▌ lower learning curve than the LAST approach; LITA/RITA dissection and anastomotic technique identical to conventional median sternotomy approach,

▌ conversion to conventional surgery with ECC is easily accomplished by extending the sternotomy; no need for patient repositioning,

▌ rapid and painless postoperative mobilization due to maintained integrity of the manubrium and sternoclavicular joint.

This is a summary of our surgical technique and our results with partial inferior sternotomy for MIDCAB procedures.

Patient selection

At this time, no absolute or general indications for MIDCAB surgery have been established. We believe that MIDCAB surgery via partial inferior sternotomy is indicated under the following clinical conditions:

▪ Patients with single vessel coronary artery disease (LAD, RCA), especially after failed PTCA or stent insertion; in addition those cases where catheter – based interventions are contraindicated (proximal or complex type C lesions),

▪ patients with multivessel coronary artery disease who become candidates for PTCA/stenting of additional vessels after surgical revascularization of the LAD (hybrid revascularization strategy),

▪ high-risk patients in whom it is advisable to minimize the surgical trauma and to avoid ECC, including patients with COPD, renal failure, severe peripheral vascular disease, and very old patients.

Intramyocardial coronary arteries, very small (< 1.5 mm), and calcified coronary arteries represent relative contraindications to MIDCAB procedures.

Surgical technique

Endotracheally intubated, supine patient under general anesthesia. Standardized monitoring including continuous cardiac output measurement with the PiCCO system (Pulsion Medical Systems, Munich, Germany) which is not affected by heart posi-

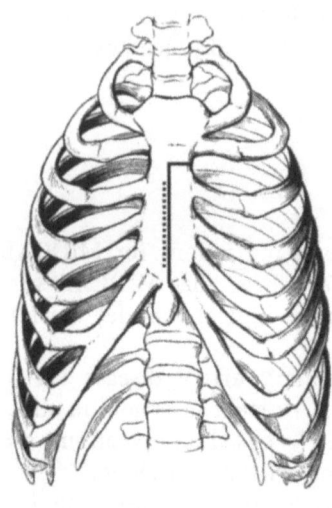

Fig. 1. Partial inferior sternotomy.
----- skin incision; ——— sternotomy

tion. Application of external defibrillator pads. Normothermia is maintained with a heating blanket and additional forced-air warming (Bair Hugger, Augustine Medical, Inc., USA).

Midline skin incision from the 3rd rib to the attachment of the xyphoid process (8–12 cm). Dissection of the left or right sternal border within the 2nd ICS. Partial transverse sternotomy at this level. Exposure is completed by extending the osteotomy longitudinally while sparing the xyphoid process (Fig. 1).

Placement of a thoracic and IMA retractor (Richard Martin Medizintechnik GmbH, Tuttlingen, Germany) or a Finochetti retractor. The ITA is first dissected off the endothoracic fascia at the cranial aspect of the vessel, thereby avoiding step forma- tion and potential damage to the vessel when the sternum is spread transversely to gain exposure. Subsequently, vascular dissection is completed, proceeding from the 1st rib proximally to the LITA/RITA bifurcation distally. The pleura does not need to be opened for this maneuver. Following systemic hepariniza- tion (150 IE/kgBW, ACT > 200 s), the LITA/RITA is divided. As an option, one can inject 2–4 ml of papaverin solution (2.5 mg/

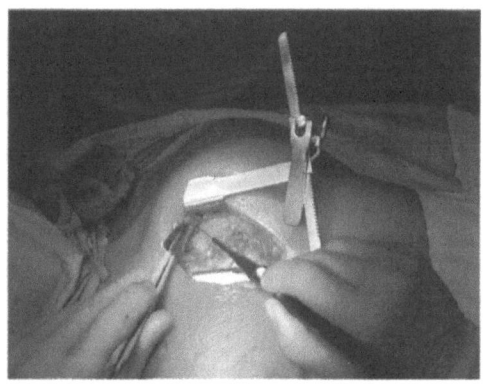

Fig. 2. LITA preparation

ml, Paveron®, Linden, Heuchelheim, Germany) into the distal end of the LITA/RITA and apply a clip to the vessel (Fig. 2).

The sternal retractor (Guidant Corporation, Cupertino, CA, USA) is inserted. After vertical pericardiotomy, right atrial and ventricular pacemaker wires are placed. AAI pacing is set at a rate of 90–100 beats/minute, thereby reducing the stroke volume while increasing cardiac output and decreasing the size of the heart. The left ventricular target vessels can be rotated to the median plane by sequential placement of pericardial traction sutures. Alternatively, a moist gauze placed behind the heart will provide exposure (Fig. 3).

The pericardium is incised laterally and the LITA/RITA pulled through the opening. Proximal to the anastomotic site, the target vessel is encircled with a vascular loop (Ethiloop, Ethicon, Brussels, Belgium). To avoid injury to the vascular endothelium distal to the anastomosis, we routinely do without a distal vessel loop. Exposure of the target vessel is achieved with the stabilizer system (Axius, Guidant Corporation, Cupertino, CA, USA). After arteriotomy, distal perfusion is carefully controlled by placing tension on the vascular loop. In cases of hemodynamic instability, arrhythmias, or pronounced signs of ischemia, an intracoronary shunt is inserted. Using a running 8-0 prolene suture, the LITA is anastomosed to the target vessel (Fig. 4).

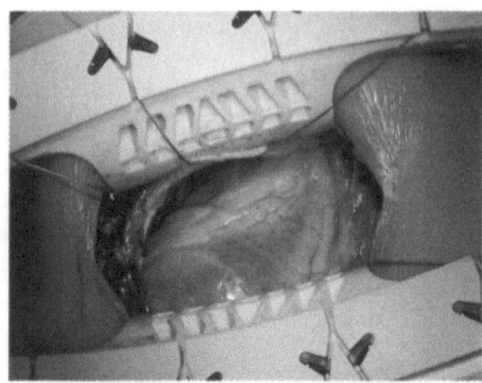

Fig. 3. LAD exposure

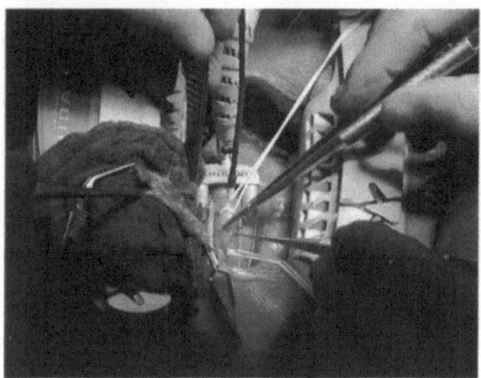

Fig. 4. Stabilization and anastomosis

After completing the anastomosis, blood flow in the native coronary artery and LITA/RITA is reopened. The LITA/RITA pedicle is secured to the epicardium with 5-0 prolene. Graft-flow is routinely measured. The pericardium is closed and a drain is inserted. The sternum is closed with two wires, the first of which is placed at an angle of approximately 45° to the longitudinal sternotomy. This technique stabilizes the transverse osteotomy (Fig. 5). The incision is closed in layers, finishing with an intradermal suture.

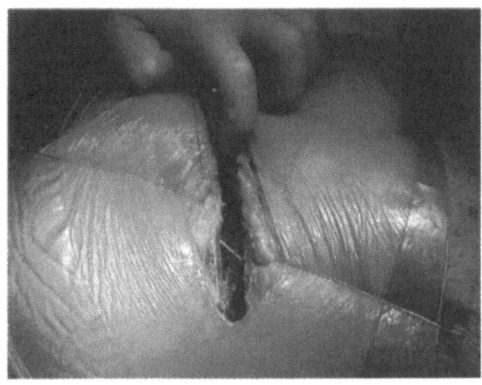

Fig. 5. Sternal closure

Clinical experience

Between December 2000 and April 2003, we performed 80 MIDCAB procedures by partial inferior sternotomy. Of our patients, 18.8% were 70 years of age or older; 40.0% of our patients had a previous myocardial infarction. LV function was impaired (EF ≤40%) in 8.8% of all patients. The preoperative patient data are summarized in Table 1.

A total of 77 patients underwent single ITA to LAD grafting. A sequential LITA to LAD/D1 graft was completed in one patient, in another, the RITA was anastomosed to the RCA. One patient underwent both LITA to LAD and RITA to RCA grafting via partial inferior sternotomy. The average operative time was 91.3 minutes (SD 19.6), the average ischemic time 6.8 minutes (SD 2.2). In two cases, the LITA was injured when the sternum was divided transversely. In the first of these cases, the LAD was revascularized with the RITA; in the second, a vein graft was utilized. Three patients (3.8%) required perioperative inotropic support. One patient, whose EF was 22%, underwent preoperative insertion of an intraaortic balloon pump (IABP); postoperative IABP placement was needed in another case. Conversion to full sternotomy or ECC was not performed in any patient. All patients survived the surgical procedure and

Table 1. Biometric and preoperative data (80 patients)

∎ Age (y)	58.9 ± 11.3
≥70 y	15 (18.8%)
∎ Female	18 (22.5%)
∎ BMI (kg/m^2)	30.1 ± 16.5
∎ Ejection fraction (%)	63.5 ± 14.1
≤40%	7 (8.8%)
∎ Previous myocardial infarction	32 (40.0%)
∎ CCS Score III or IV	14 (17.5%)
∎ Unstable angina	14 (17.5%)
∎ Diabetes	23 (28.8%)
∎ Hypertension	69 (86.3%)
∎ Renal failure	4 (5.0%)
∎ COPD	12 (15.0%)

BMI body mass index, *CCS* Canadian Cardiovascular Society, *COPD* chronic obstructive pulmonary disease. Values are mean ± SD or number (percentage)

Table 2. Perioperative data (80 patients)

∎ Grafts	
LAD	77
LAD + D1	1
RCA	1
RCA + LAD	1
∎ Ischemic (occlusion) time (min)	6.8 ± 2.2
∎ Operative time (min)	91.3 ± 19.6
∎ Graft flow (ml)	31.3 ± 21.7
∎ Use of inotropes	3 (3.8%)
∎ Number of patient transfused	2 (2.5%)
∎ IABP postoperative	2 (2.5%)
∎ Conversion (full sternotomy or ECC)	0

IABP intraaortic balloon pump, *ECC* extracorporeal circulation. Values are mean ± SD or number (percentage) were transferred to the intensive care unit in stable condition. The perioperative data are summarized in Table 2.

Postoperative results and clinical outcome are presented in Table 3. On the first postoperative day, the overwhelming majority of patients (61.3%) were transferred to the regular ward. A total of 45% of patients were artificially ventilated for 6 hours or less. During the initial 18 hours, tube drainage averaged 468.2 ml (SD 429.7). The rate of re-thoracotomies was 6.3%. None of the patients suffered a perioperative myocardial infarction or stroke. Throughout the postoperative course, sternal wound infections were detected in 5% of patients. One female patient died 43 days postoperatively from septic multiorgan failure as a result of mediastinitis. In addition to reduced ventricular function, her comorbidities included a body mass index of 42.4 kg/m^2, insulin-dependent diabetes mellitus, and renal failure.

Table 3. Postoperative data (80 patients)

▌ Time on ventilator (h)	8.2 ± 5.9
≤6 h	36 (45.0%)
▌ Duration of ICU stay (h)	35.2 ± 29.1
≤24 h	49 (61.3%)
▌ Blood loss (ml/18 h)	468.2 ± 429.7
▌ Number of patient transfused	5 (6.3%)
▌ Re-exploration for bleeding	5 (6.3%)
▌ Wound infection	4 (5.0%)
▌ Pneumonia	0
▌ Stroke	0
▌ Atrial fibrillation	17 (21.3%)
▌ Peak serum CK (μmol/ls)	6.8 ± 6.3
▌ Peak serum CK-MB (μmol/ls)	0.51 ± 0.59
▌ Mortality	
≤30 days	0
>30 days	1 (1.3%)

ICU intensive care unit. Values are mean ± SD or number (percentage)

Summary

MIDCAB via partial inferior sternotomy is an effective and safe approach for surgical revascularization of anterior wall coronary arteries and the RCA. In our view, the procedure is indicated in patients with single or double vessel coronary artery disease, especially after failed interventional therapy. As elucidated in the introduction, partial inferior sternotomy has several advantages compared to the LAST approach. The cosmetic results are similar. In addition, the method deserves special attention for high-risk cases.

References

1. Acuff TE, Landreneau RJ, Griffith BP, Mack MJ (1996) Minimally invasive coronary artery bypass grafting. Ann Thorac Surg 61(1):135–137
2. Arom KV, Emery RW, Nicoloff DM (1996) Mini-sternotomy for coronary artery bypass grafting. Ann Thorac Surg 61(4):1271–1272
3. Bauer M, Pasic M, Ewert R, Hetzer R (2001) Ministernotomy versus complete sternotomy for coronary bypass operations: no difference in postoperative pulmonary function. J Thorac Cardiovasc Surg 121(4):702–707
4. Benetti FJ, Ballester C (1995) Use of thoracoscopy and a minimal thoracotomy, in mammary-coronary bypass to left anterior descending artery, without extracorporeal circulation. Experience in 2 cases. J Cardiovasc Surg (Torino) 36(2):159–161
5. Calafiore AM, Di Giammarco G, Teodori G, Gallina S, Maddestra N, Paloscia L, et al (1998) Midterm results after minimally invasive coronary surgery (LAST operation). J Thorac Cardiovasc Surg 115(4):763–771
6. Detter C, Reichenspurner H, Bochm DH, Thalhammer M, Schutz A, Reichart B (2001) Single vessel revascularization with beating heart techniques – minithoracotomy or sternotomy? Eur J Cardiothorac Surg 19(4):464–470

7. Diegeler A, Thiele H, Falk V, Hambrecht R, Spyrantis N, Sick P, et al (2002) Comparison of stenting with minimally invasive bypass surgery for stenosis of the left anterior descending coronary artery. N Engl J Med 347(8):561–566

8. Goy JJ, Eeckhout E, Moret C, Burnand B, Vogt P, Stauffer JC, et al (1999) Five-year outcome in patients with isolated proximal left anterior descending coronary artery stenosis treated by angioplasty or left internal mammary artery grafting. A prospective trial. Circulation 99(25):3255–3259

9. Goy JJ, Kaufmann U, Goy-Eggenberger D, Garachemani A, Hurni M, Carrel T, et al (2000) A prospective randomized trial comparing stenting to internal mammary artery grafting for proximal, isolated de novo left anterior coronary artery stenosis: the SIMA trial. Stenting vs Internal Mammary Artery. Mayo Clin Proc 75(11):1116–1123

10. Hueb WA, Bellotti G, de Oliveira SA, Arie S, de Albuquerque CP, Jatene AD, et al (1995) The Medicine, Angioplasty or Surgery Study (MASS): a prospective, randomized trial of medical therapy, balloon angioplasty or bypass surgery for single proximal left anterior descending artery stenoses. J Am Coll Cardiol 26(7):1600–1605

11. Izzat MB, Yim AP, El-Zufari MH, Khaw KS (1998) Upper T ministernotomy for aortic valve operations. Chest 114(1):291–294

12. Kolessov VI (1967) Mammary artery-coronary artery anastomosis as method of treatment for angina pectoris. J Thorac Cardiovasc Surg 54(4):535–544

13. Loop FD (1996) Internal-thoracic-artery grafts. Biologically better coronary arteries. N Engl J Med 334(4):263–265

14. Loop FD, Lytle BW, Cosgrove DM, Stewart RW, Goormastic M, Williams GW, et al (1986) Influence of the internal-mammary-artery graft on 10-year survival and other cardiac events. N Engl J Med 314(1):1–6

15. Moreno-Cabral RJ (1997) Mini-T sternotomy for cardiac operations. J Thorac Cardiovasc Surg 113(4):810–811

16. Robinson MC, Gross DR, Zeman W, Stedje-Larsen E (1995) Minimally invasive coronary artery bypass grafting: a new method using an anterior mediastinotomy. J Card Surg 10(5):529–536

17. Subramanian VA (1996) Clinical experience with minimally invasive reoperative coronary bypass surgery. Eur J Cardiothorac Surg 10(12):1058–1062

18. Trehan N, Malhotra R, Mishra Y, Shrivastva S, Kohli V, Mehta Y
(2000) Comparison of ministernotomy with minithoracotomy regarding postoperative pain and internal mammary artery characteristics. Heart Surg Forum 3(4):300–306
19. Walterbusch G (1998) Partial sternotomy for cardiac operations. J
Thorac Cardiovasc Surg 115(1):256–258

Robotic-enhanced MIDCAB

C. Detter, D. Böhm

Introduction

Minimally invasive direct coronary artery bypass grafting (MIDCAB) through a small anterior minithoracotomy for single-vessel revascularization to the left anterior descending coronary artery (LAD) have been introduced as an alternative to standard coronary artery bypass grafting and have become widely employed [3, 14]. For further improvement in patient outcome, new clinical pathways have emerged [5]. With an endoscopic approach using robotic-enhanced surgery, the surgical trauma can be minimized. Endoscopic techniques allows complete and atraumatic mobilization of the internal mammary artery (IMA) with a small amount of chest wall trauma. Thus, no spreading of the rib cage or removal of ribs is required, reducing postoperative pain and improving patient satisfaction.

This chapter describes an endoscopic atraumatic procedure combined with standard MIDCAB techniques using robotic-enhanced surgery.

Endoscopic atraumatic coronary artery bypass

The endoscopic atraumatic coronary artery bypass (Endo-ACAB) technique consists of endoscopic IMA harvesting followed by an atraumatic small chest incision. In this procedure, a robotic arm is used to assist the surgeon in endoscopic IMA harvesting.

A double-lumen endotracheal tube for intermittent single-lung ventilation is used routinely during the operation. The patient is placed in a supine position with the left side of the chest slightly elevated (approximately 20 degrees) and the left arm raised and fixed above the patient's head. This provides more room for the right-handed endoscopic instrument. To avoid brachial plexus palsy, it is extremely important to pad and support the scapula. After deflation of the left lung, three lateral thoracic ports were inserted in the third, fifth and seventh intercostal space (ICS). The camera port in the fifth ICS is inserted at the level of the anterior axillary line, the instrument port for a grasper or endoscopic Kittner at the seventh ICS slightly more anterior, and the cautery at the third or fourth ICS in the anterior axillary line for dissection of the superior or inferior portions of the IMA (Fig. 1). Continuous carbon dioxide insufflation at levels of 8 to 10 mmHg is used to optimize visualization. This is absolutely necessary in providing the space needed to harvest the entire length of the left IMA from the subclavian artery down to the bifurcation at the level of the sixth rib. IMA harvesting can be performed with electrocautery (Genzyme Surgical, Cambridge, MA) or the Harmonic Scalpel® (Ethicon EndoSurgery, Inc, Somerville, NJ). Using cautery, a long cautery extension coupled with a smoke evacuator is used. The cautery setting is kept low (20–30 Watts) to avoid thermal injury to the IMA and splattering of the scope lens. A clear and dry field should be maintained because bleeding can obscure the view significantly. With the Harmonic Scalpel®, the likelihood of injury to the IMA is lessened. Thus, we prefer the Harmonic Scalpel® for IMA harvesting. To avoid obscuring the view which can be caused by excessive aerosolized particles within the chest cavity, a needle should be placed in the chest on low suction. The IMA is harvested totally endoscopic with robotic visualization. The robotic arm (AESOP®, Computer Motion Inc., Goleta, CA) is placed opposite the surgeon and is used to hold the endoscope and to control its posi-

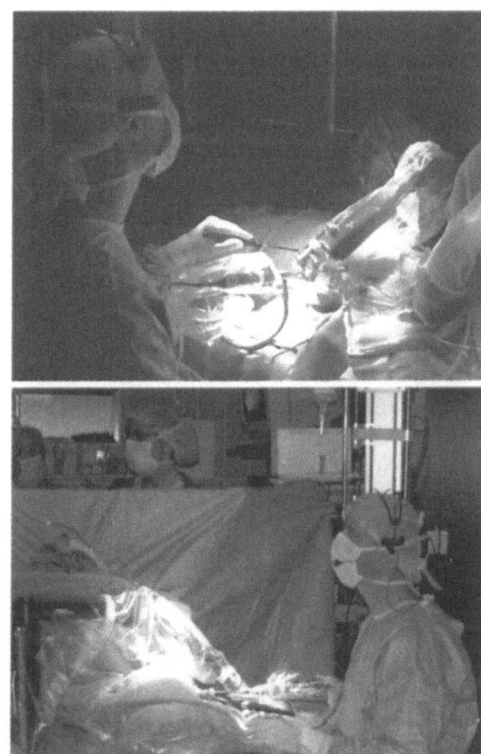

Fig. 1. Endoscopic IMA harvesting. The voice-activated AESOP® robotic arm is used to hold and to control the endoscope

tion via simple voice commands by the surgeon. This allows for greater precision, stability, and efficiency than can be achieved with direct human control, facilitating endoscopic procedures.

After harvesting of the IMA, the pericardium is endoscopically opened. The target vessel is identified and the coronary anatomy is evaluated. At this stage, the procedure can easily be switched to a sternotomy approach due to a heavily calcified or very small vessel. Without opening of the chest wall, the surgeon is able to endoscopically detect and locate the optimal target area for coronary anastomosis. To verify the ideal location of the incision, a spinal needle is placed through the anterior chest wall over this site. Thus, a small lateral incision can be made directly over the target area. The pectoralis muscle is separated and care is taken not to spread the ribs. This minimizes patient trauma and scarring, and avoids the significant pain associated with rib spreading. A small MIDCAB retractor or a soft tissue retractor is used for exposure of the operative site.

To achieve local immobilization of the target vessel, a mechanical pressure stabilizer (CTS MIDCAB stabilizer; Cardio-Thoracic Systems Inc, Cupertino, CA) or the platform technique (Genzyme MIDCAB stabilizer with Cohn platform; Genzyme Surgical Products, Fall River, MA) can be used. Alternatively, an endoscopic stabilizer (Computer Motion Inc., Goleta, CA) can be inserted through the scope port incision. Using an endoscopic stabilizer, only the instruments go through the incision to minimize the need to retract the ribs.

The coronary artery is surrounded proximally to the region of the anastomosis with 4-0 or 5-0 polypropylene sutures (Ethicon, Somerville, NJ) that is snared over a pledget for temporary interruption of blood flow or with silastic tapes to achieve hemostasis. The anastomosis between the LIMA and the LAD is manually performed on the beating heart with a single 7-0 or 8-0 polypropylene running suture (Ethicon, Somerville, NJ) using conventional instruments under direct vision. A humidified carbon dioxide blower is employed to clear blood from the operative field.

Intraoperative quality assessment should be performed using ultrasound-based flow meters. An intercostal block of 0.5% Bupivacain is administered. A small chest tube is placed through the scope port incision.

▌ Robotic-enhanced MIDCAB

Alternatively, a robotic system can be used for robotic-enhanced, totally endoscopic IMA harvesting. This technique allows a safe harvesting of the left or right IMA, or both, via three left lateral ports, followed by a manually performed LIMA-LAD anastomosis through a MIDCAB incision (Robotic-enhanced MIDCAB).

The two robotic microsurgical systems that are presently under clinical investigation are the ZEUS® Robotic Surgical System (Computer Motion Inc., Goleta, CA) and the da VINCI™ telemanipulation system (Intuitive Surgical, Inc., Mountain View, CA). Both systems enable the surgeon to manipulate instruments in real-time on a remote operative field, linked by the computer system, and have been used to perform endoscopic CABG [2, 8, 10, 12]. The computer controller performs natural tremor filtration and scales instrument movements to different ratios. The surgeon's hand movements at the console are scaled down and filtered into precise micro-movements at the operative site. 3-D visualization systems are included to sufficiently visualize spatial orientation of the vessel and instrument position. The combination of robotics and 3-D visualization creates depth perception and enhances speed and safety.

▌ Endoscopic IMA harvesting using the ZEUS® Robotic System

The ZEUS® Robotic Surgical System with MicroWrist™ consists of three principal components: an ergonomically enhanced surgeon console, a computer control system, and three interactive, table-mounted robotic arms (Fig. 2a,b). One robotic arm (AESOP®, Computer Motion Inc.) is used to hold the endoscope and to control its position via simple voice commands. The other two robotic arms manipulate surgical instruments under the surgeon's remote control. The surgeon console con-

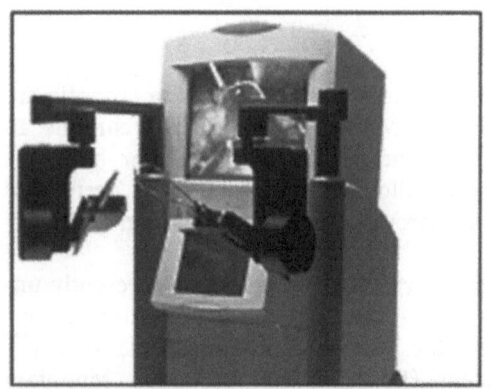

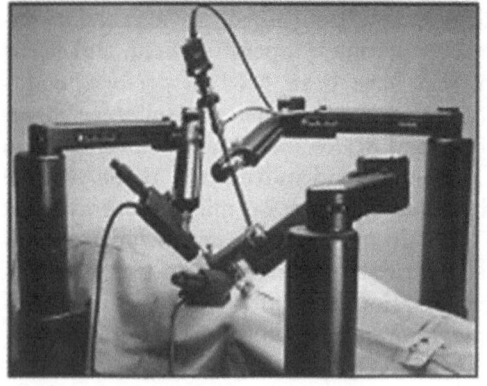

Fig. 2. The ZEUS® Robotic Surgical System consists of three principal components: an ergonomically enhanced surgeon console (**a**), a computer control system, and three interactive, table-mounted robotic arms (**b**)

sists of a video monitor and two instrument handles. Movements of the surgical instruments are controlled by form-fitted handles. These are scaled and tremor is filtered to perform fully endoscopic and accurate microsurgery.

The operative setting is similar to the Endo-ACAB technique using a double lumen tube and single lung ventilation. The patient is in a supine position with 30° left chest elevation, and the left arm elevated to avoid external robotic arm collisions.

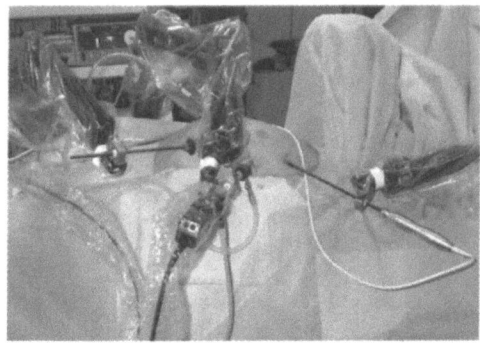

Fig. 3. Endoscopic IMA harvesting using the ZEUS® robotic telemanipulation system and the Harmonic Scalpel®

After deflation of the left lung, three lateral thoracic ports are inserted in the third, fifth and seventh ICS. During the procedure, carbon dioxide gas is insufflated into the pleural cavity up to a pressure of 5 to 10 mmHg. A 5 mm 30-degree endoscope is first placed through the insufflation port in the fifth ICS at the level of the anterior axillary line and adapted to the voice-activated AESOP® robotic arm. A second 5 mm port is inserted in the third ICS in the mid-axillary line for the Harmonic Scalpel, which is attached to the right robotic arm. A third 5 mm port is placed in the seventh ICS in the mid-axillary line for a Kittner dissector (Ethicon EndoSurgery, Inc, Somerville, NJ) or forceps, which is attached to the left robotic arm (Fig. 3). A proper positioning of the patient with the left arm elevated and the distances between the ports are essential.

IMA harvesting is performed while the surgeon is sitting at the console by moving the instruments with handles and controlling the endoscope with voice commands. With the Harmonic Scalpel® side branches can be transected with excellent hemostasis without using hemoclips. The Kittner dissector is used to provide gentle counter traction during the dissection.

After complete harvesting of the IMA, the pericardium is endoscopically opened and the target coronary vessel is identified.

The robotic system is removed and the anastomosis is manually performed directly through a small MIDCAB incision as described above.

Conclusions

New surgical techniques for the treatment of the isolated lesion of the LAD include MIDCAB surgery and endoscopic harvesting of the IMA with or without the use of a robotic-enhanced system. Endoscopic IMA harvesting has become an integral part of MIDCAB procedures [9, 11, 18]. This technique minimizes the surgical trauma associated with rib spreading and chest wall retraction during direct-vision IMA harvest through the anterior minithoracotomy [16]. Endoscopic harvesting of the IMA avoids these hazards. It allows complete dissection from the subclavian artery down to the sixth rib without any traumatic retraction, thus, reducing postoperative pain and patient discomfort.

The atraumatic coronary artery bypass (Endo-ACAB) technique consists of an endoscopic IMA harvesting followed by an atraumatic chest incision through which a direct-vision anastomosis is performed using conventional instruments. The Endo-ACAB overcomes the tremendous shortcomings of the MIDCAB procedure and provides superior outcomes [15]. The key elements of making this procedure atraumatic are 1) reducing the surgical and CPB-related trauma and 2) avoiding rib-spreading and disruption of the bony chest wall, thus, limiting stress on the thoracic skeleton and minimizing postoperative pain. This reduces patient discomfort and allows faster patient recovery with faster return to normal activity.

The introduction of robotic-enhanced surgery enables the development of new endoscopic procedures, demanding a stepwise approach [4, 7]. Initially, a robotic surgical system can be used for harvesting the IMA, followed by a manually performed anastomosis through a small lateral minithoracotomy (robotic-enhanced MIDCAB). This is a step towards a total endoscopic CABG with the use of a computer-enhanced surgical robotic system. The application of a robotic-enhanced endoscopic method allows a safe and complete harvesting of the left or right IMA, or both [7]. The high-magnification visualization, as well as the scaled instrument manipulation enabled the dissection of a thin vascular pedicle without injuring adjacent structures. The advantage of robotic surgery arises from the capability to have intrathoracically five or six degrees freedom of motion and an optimized 3-D visualization. The integrated computer between the instrument handle and instrument tip eliminates the high-frequency tremor movements and enhances dexterity through motion-scaling.

However, endoscopic and robotic-enhanced MIDCAB is limited to the vessels of the anterior and anterolateral wall. To overcome these limitations, the concept of endoscopic and robotic-enhanced MIDCAB can be combined with catheter-based procedures like percutaneous coronary angioplasty and stenting, allowing complete revascularization for multivessel coronary artery disease [1, 6, 17]. This hybrid procedure accomplishes the goal of complete revascularization with an LIMA-LAD graft while minimizing surgical trauma and lowering risk [13].

References

1. Amodeo VJ, Donias HW, Dancona G, Hoover EL, Karamanoukian HL (2002) The hybrid approach to coronary artery revascularization: minimally invasive direct coronary artery bypass with percutaneous coronary intervention. Angiology 53:665–669
2. Boyd WD, Rayman R, Desai ND, Menkis AH, Dobkowski W, Ganapathy S, Kiaii B, Jablonsky G, McKenzie FN, Novick RJ (2000) Closed-chest coronary artery bypass grafting on the beating heart with the use of a computer-enhanced surgical robotic system. J Thorac Cardiovasc Surg 120:807–809

3. Calafiore AM, Giammarco GD, Teodori G, Bosco G, D'Annunzio E, Barsotti A, Maddestra N, Paloscia L, Vitolla G, Sciarra A, Fino C, Contini M (1996) Left anterior descending coronary artery grafting via left anterior small thoracotomy without cardiopulmonary bypass. Ann Thorac Surg 61:1658–1665

4. Detter C, Boehm DH, Reichenspurner H, Deuse T, Arnold M, Reichart B (2002) Robotically-assisted coronary artery surgery with and without cardiopulmonary bypass – from first clinical use to endoscopic operation. Med Sci Monit 8:118–123

5. Diegeler A (1999) Left internal mammary artery grafting to left anterior descending coronary artery by minimally invasive direct coronary artery bypass approach. Curr Cardiol Rep 1:323–330

6. Friedrich GJ, Bonatti J, Dapunt OE (1997) Preliminary experience with minimally invasive coronary-artery bypass surgery combined with coronary angioplasty. N Engl J Med 336:1454–1455

7. Kappert U, Schneider J, Cichon R, Gulielmos V, Tugtekin SM, Nicolai J, Matschke K, Schueler S (2001) Development of robotic enhanced endoscopic surgery for the treatment of coronary artery disease. Circulation 104(12 Suppl 1):I102–107

8. Loulmet D, Carpentier A, d'Attellis N, Berrebi A, Cardon C, Ponzio O, Aupecle B, Relland JY (1999) Endoscopic coronary artery bypass grafting with the aid of robotic assisted instruments. J Thorac Cardiovasc Surg 118:4–10

9. Mack MJ, Acuff T, Osborne J (1998) Minimally invasive direct coronary artery bypass: technical considerations and instrumentation. J Card Surg 13:290–296

10. Mohr FW, Falk V, Diegeler A, Walther T, Gummert JF, Bucerius J, Jacobs S, Autschbach R (2001) Computer-enhanced "robotic" cardiac surgery: experience in 148 patients. J Thorac Cardiovasc Surg 121:842–853

11. Nataf P, Al-Attar N, Ramadan R, Scorcin M, Raffoul R, Salvi S, Lessana A (2000) Thoracoscopic IMA takedown. J Card Surg 15:278–282

12. Reichenspurner H, Damiano RJ, Mack M, Boehm DH, Gulbins H, Detter C, Meiser B, Ellgass R, Reichart B (1999) Use of the voice-controlled and computer-assisted surgical system ZEUS for endoscopic coronary artery bypass grafting. J Thorac Cardiovasc Surg 118:11–16

13. Stahl KD, Boyd WD, Vassiliades TA, Karamanoukian HL (2002) Hybrid robotic coronary artery surgery and angioplasty in multivessel coronary artery disease. Ann Thorac Surg 74:S1358–1362

14. Subramanian VA, McCabe JC, Geller CM (1997) Minimally invasive direct coronary artery bypass grafting: two-year clinical experience. Ann Thorac Surg 64:1648–1655

15. Vassiliades TA Jr (2002) Technical aids to performing thoracoscopic robotically-assisted internal mammary artery harvesting. Heart Surg Forum 5:119–124

16. Vassiliades TA Jr (2001) Atraumatic coronary artery bypass (ACAB): techniques and outcome. Heart Surg Forum 4:331–334

17. Wittwer T, Cremer J, Boonstra P, Grandjean J, Mariani M, Mugge A, Drexler H, den Heijer P, Leitner ER, Hepp A, Wehr M, Haverich A (2000) Myocardial "hybrid" revascularisation with minimally invasive direct coronary artery bypass grafting combined with coronary angioplasty: preliminary results of a multicentre study. Heart 83:58–63

18. Wolf RK, Ohtsuka T, Flege JB Jr (1998) Early results of thoracoscopic internal mammary artery harvest using an ultrasonic scalpel. Eur J Cardiothorac Surg 14:S54–57

Off-pump totally endoscopic coronary artery bypass grafting

U. Kappert, J. Schneider, S. M. Tugtekin

Introduction

In the thrive towards a minimization of access in minimally invasive cardiac surgery, wrist-enhanced robotic instrumentation is currently leading to a turning point in the history of minimally invasive cardiac surgery as totally endoscopic coronary artery bypass grafting procedures become feasible [1, 4–6, 9, 10, 12, 17].

An endoscopic technique recently in use for the revascularization of single vessel coronary artery disease (left anterior descending artery – LAD) can be seen as a result of an ongoing technical evolution. It serves as a fine example of how heart surgery has changed and progressed during the past eight years.

Based on the conventional standards in coronary artery surgery, a concept of minimally invasive revascularization was started in 1996. Initial steps for an endoscopic cardiac operation were complicated due to the rigidity of the two dimensional-based instrumentation. As a consequence handling proved difficult. A further aspect was limited space inside the chest.

Classical endoscopic instrumentation carries certain disadvantages, especially lack of wrist enhancement and 3-D visualization. The development of a robotic system, consisting of a master-slave construction, led to the development of an advanced endoscopic telemanipulatory system with full clinical use in 1998.

Beside this, due to the application of a technically refined computer-based operating unit endoscopically bypass operations became a reality [1, 14, 18].

As a matter of fact, the development of endoscopic instrumentation imitating the movement of the human hand with all its degrees of freedom of motion has become a breakthrough in cardiac surgery.

After the introduction of a special endostabilizer in 2001, patient selection for an endoscopic cardiac operation has been extended to off-pump procedures. This new technical feature in minimally invasive cardiac surgery enables TECAB procedures for coronary artery disease using 4 stab incisions even on the beating heart [5, 6, 9, 15].

In this section, we focus on surgery for the endoscopic myocardial revascularization on the beating heart.

Patient selection

At present, isolated stenosis of the proximal left anterior descending coronary artery is currently the domain of PTCA. On the other hand, current studies have shown evidence for high efficiency of surgery for this particular patient group [8, 16].

In surgical patients, a significantly lower reintervention rate (37 vs. 3%) was showen. Within the frame of the above studies, single vessel coronary artery disease should not be considered an indication for cardiologic intervention.

Additionally Diegeler et al. [2] revealed in a prospective study comparing the outcome after PTCA or surgery for isolated stenosis of the LAD, a significantly lower reintervention rate in the surgical group.

Due to the promising results, the surgical therapy for proximal high grade LAD stenosis in this patient group receive particular interest for the use of minimally invasive surgical techniques. Our concept for minimally invasive surgery is directed to develop a safe and efficient approach with low perioperative morbidity in this highly selected patient group offering a true or even superior alternative to PTCA.

Angiography has a key role for adequate patients selection for operative endoscopic myocardial intervention. Currently, the indication for this kind of operation represents a type A lesion of the LAD (length below 10 mm, concentric vessel, even vessel endothelium, easy access, angled below 45°, low amount of calcification, far from the ostium, no thrombus).

Exclusion criteria were decreased left ventricular ejection fraction (LVEF <40%), impaired lung function (FEV1 <1.0 L), pleural and pericardial adhesions, reoperation, obesity (body mass index >35 kg/m^2), intramyocardial LAD course and diffuse coronary artery sclerosis.

Definitive evaluation and prediction of these contraindications are sometimes not possible and therefore the decision for the totally endoscopically procedure can only be made intraoperatively and must fit to the individual circumstances of each patient. In our own experience with 56 TECAB procedures, the conversion rate to the MIDCAB procedure was still quite high [9]. This is definitely related to missing diagnostic evaluation of the morphology and anatomy of the LAD.

In the future, further diagnostic methods should be available for a better preoperative evaluation of each patient. Adequate preoperative evaluation should help the surgeon to predict whether a patient is suitable for a TECAB procedure or should primarily undergo a MIDCAB or even median sternotomy.

Surgical technique

The computer-based robotic system (da Vinci^{TM}, Intuitive Surgical, Mountain View, CA, USA) is described in detail in the literature [1, 12, 14]. The patient is placed in the supine position with the left arm resting slightly beneath the posterior axillary line. After induction of general anesthesia a double lumen tube or a endotracheal blocker is used for single-lung ventilation during surgery.

Further aspects of anesthesia management are discussed in another chapter.

▌ Placement of the Ports

The three 1-cm skin incisions are placed in the left chest in the 3rd intercostal space (ICS) at the medioclavicular line for the right port, in the 5th ICS at the anterior axillary line for the central optical port and in the 6th ICS at the medioclavicular line for the left port forming a triangle whose angle may vary depending on the habitus of the patient (Fig. 1).

One of the simple rules for a correct port placement is the establishment of an even equilateral triangle. Before the introduction of the camera port, single lung ventilation should have been started for at least 2–3 min. This is essential, as the non-ventilated lung needs some time to collapse, thus, avoiding injury the lung. After this, the ports can be introduced into the pleura at a lower risk of perforation injury. Then, through the camera port, warmed and humidified CO_2 insufflation is started at pressures between 5 and 10 mmHg. The camera system is then introduced via this central port.

Following a brief exploration of the left chest cavity and identification of the LIMA, the slave unit of the da Vinci^{TM} surgical system is placed to the right of the patient and the two other ports are introduced.

For the right instrument, the median between left nipple and left shoulder seems to be the best position for its introduction. The left instrument can be placed best at a point where the left ventricular apex is expected. Misplaced ports can make performance of a TECAB procedure impossible and make MIDCAB necessary.

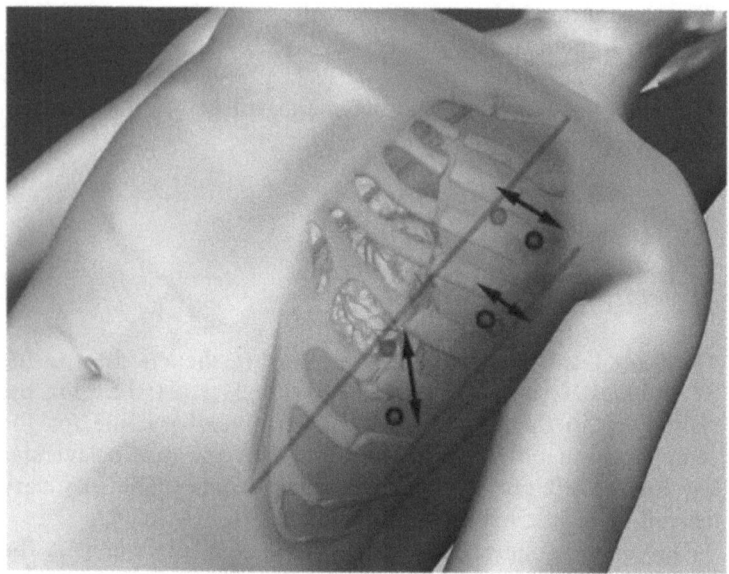

Fig. 1. The three 1-cm skin incisions are placed in the left chest in the 3rd intercostal space (ICS) at the medioclavicular line for the right port, in the 5th ICS at the anterior axillary line for the central optical port and in the 6th ICS at the medioclavicular line for the left port forming a triangle whose angle may vary depending on the habitus of the patient

LIMA takedown

A slight upward movement of the camera port under CO_2 insufflation improves IMA dissection due to increase of the precordial space, which is essential for IMA takedown and LAD grafting. Using 30 Watts cautery, endoscopic LIMA takedown is begun creating a pedicle.

In the distal area (2 cm), the mammary artery is skeletonized in order to facilitate the coronary anastomosis. After IMA harvesting an appropriate bulldog clamp is introduced via the skin incision at the level of the 3rd ICS and is placed on the proximal IMA. Heparin is administered in order to achieve an ACT (anticoagulation time) longer than 300 s.

For this operative step it is necessary to take out the right instrument. Via the same incision the vessel clamp being attached to a thread is placed at the proximal IMA by endoscopic means.

This procedural step has two advantages. On one hand, the IMA needs not be prepared in this area and, on the other hand, there is more working space available for the procurement of the coronary anastomosis. A potential disadvantage is a larger trauma of the intercostal space as the right port is reinstalled at the same location, which in some cases proves difficult to perform.

The pericardial fat is then dissected as a flap to the left lateral aspects of the pericardium and the latter is opened in a rectangular fashion exposing the LAD. Identification of the LAD may be become difficult in the setting of large diagonal branches. In this case, exact knowledge of coronary morphology is essential to avoid malinsertion. The distal branches of the mammary artery are coagulated. The IMA is prepared for anastomosis in a usual manner and then incised longitudinally on a length of approximately 6 to 7 mm. The endo Pott's scissors is also used as a ruler. Now the IMA is ready for anastomosis.

The fourth port

Via a further fourth, 1 cm skin incision at the subxyphoidal area the endoscopic stabilizer is introduced. The right point of insertion is the end of the distal IMA close to the arch of the ribs. Using this landmark a correct positioning of the endostabilizer is secured.

In obese patients the installation can be difficult as the length of the port is limited. A procedural step – the removal of mediastinal fat up to the diaphragm from the inside should enable the introduction. This furthermore facilitates the introduction of vessel loops and suture material into the chest of the patient.

After the port has been properly installed, vessel loops are introduced. The loops are sized to approximately 10 cm from each other. A special needle holder has proved best for their introduction through the port. One of the loops is placed proximal to the planned area of anastomosis and the other one distally.

The sutures (7/0 prolene) follow via the fourth port. One of them is attached in proximity to the sternum and serves as a backup suture. With the second suture the first stitch through the IMA is made while IMA is not totally divided.

The next step is the introduction, placement and positioning of the endoscopic stabilizer. Different techniques can be applied depending on the stabilizer used and its fixation at the operating table.

Endoscopic Stabilizer

For this operating technique, a special designed endostabilizer is imperative. Various teams have operated using this technique and concluded that some changes and modifications have to be made regarding the device in order to secure a proper and reliable functioning.

Concerning our experience the second generation tool seems to be most appropriate for this most demanding type of endoscopic surgery (Fig. 2). This endoscopic device consists of two branches like common beating heart stabilizers. The branches can be guided from outside the chest. A joint at the heel of the stabilizing device allows a precise and stable positioning at the anastomotic site.

For the attachment of silastic vessel loops, for coronary occlusion, the branches of the coronary stabilizer carry special cleats

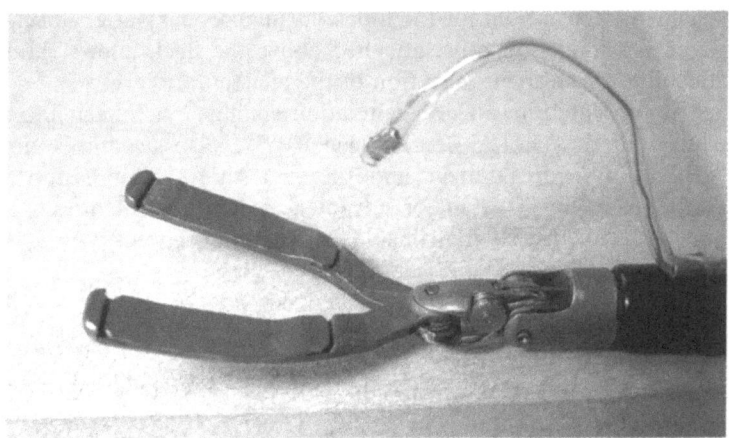

Fig. 2. Endoscopic stabilizer (second generation)

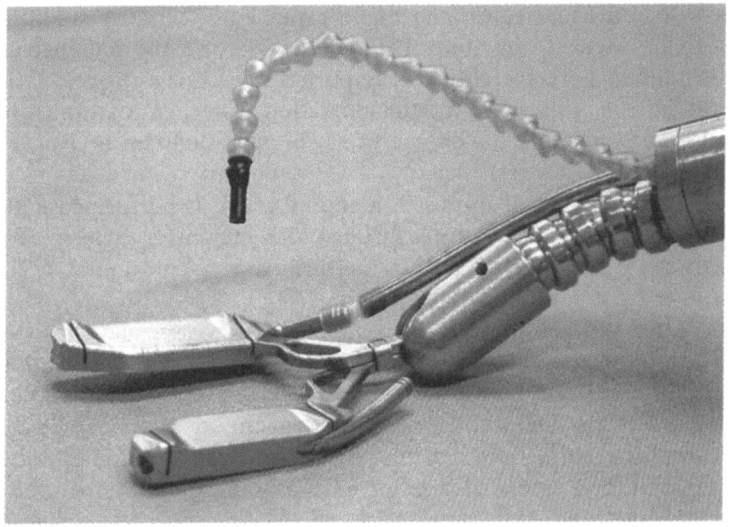

Fig. 3. Endoscopic stabilizer (third generation)

ensuring a firm hold for the loops during coronary artery occlusion. An irrigation tube, attached above the heel, allows saline flushing for clear visualization of the anastomotic area.

At present time a third generation stabilizer has been introduced in the clinical setting (Fig. 3). We also used this new generation endostabilizer and the first clinical impression is very promising. One major advantage is the placement can be easily performed by the console surgeon endoscopically.

Endoscopic anastomosis

Starting with the beaver blade, the LAD is eased from surrounding tissue and then occluded using the vessel loops. The LAD is incised with a 15 degree stitch scalpel.

Once the arteriotomy is made using Pott's scissors, a shunt can be used at any time. For delivery, we use the left instrumentation port. Hereby, it is important to avoid a drop of CO_2 pressure at this point of the operation! The loss of exposure can be costly, and the course of a safe operation can be jeopardized.

After opening of the LAD, a second stitch is performed with the already placed suture through the mammary artery. The coronary anastomosis is then performed in a continuous fashion using a running suture.

After the anastomosis is completed, the vessel clamp is released and the anastomosis is explored for leakage. Protamine is administered, and the actuators and camera are removed. After the ports are deployed from the patient the incisions should be carefully examined for bleeding. The insertion of a soft chest tube through the 1 cm incision in the 6th ICS in combination with subcutaneous and skin sutures completes the procedure. Before transferal of the patient to the intensive care unit, a single lumen endotracheal tube replaces the double lumen endotracheal tube or the endotracheal blocker is simply removed.

Comment

The technical development of an endoscopic stabilizer (Intuitive Surgical, Mountain View, CA, USA) led to a beating-heart closed-chest procedure via four 1-cm chest incisions. With the demonstrated surgical technique at hand, an optional new concept for the minimally invasive surgical treatment of CAD can be developed [10].

Many factors still influence the performance of this kind of delicate surgery; hence high conversion rates to other minimally invasive techniques or median sternotomy still occur.

The conversion rate to a MIDCAB procedure (33.9%) may decline in the future by growing experience with this new endoscopic technique. Further technical improvements concerning LAD occlusion, endoscopic stabilization and better LAD identification may lead to overcome the present obstacles.

A mature, standard regarding procedural steps should be used by the team. Too many new innovations, constantly changing new stabilizers, different suture material, new ways of performing the anastomosis and new autosuture devices as well as too few operations performed by the team reduce outcome of surgery. The development of a safe standard is essential and ongoing at present, regarding the performance of myocardial revascularization on the beating heart avoiding thoracotomy completely.

At our institution, two teams were chosen to perform these interventions, consisting of two surgeons at the console, two assisting surgeons, a perfusiologist and a team of anesthesiologists.

Currently, robotic surgery with this system should still only be performed by a few teams, as a learning curve is associated with the use of the system and the difficulties concerning communication and coordination account for it.

As described above, proper port placement setup plays an essential role in this endoscopic bypass procedure. The robotic arm placement setup is paramount to reducing the degree of difficulty and ensuring the success of the procedure. The previously postulated rule of creating a triangle-like port arrangement in the left chest of the patient is not always reliable to ensure a safe case. Modifications have to take place in accordance with the patient habitus.

Using experience and intuition, the surgeon will create an arrangement which is suitable for ensuring proper instrumentation movement inside and outside the chest by a careful evaluation of the patient intercostal spaces, rib cage, body mass index, breast size and tissue rigidity. The ports have to be moved according to these factors to avoid actuator collisions.

Our early experiences with this procedure as an essential alternative to conventional heart surgery are positive and represent only the first steps towards future developments. Closed chest off-pump coronary artery bypass grafting of single vessel coronary artery disease was performed using the da Vinci^{TM} surgical system. This new minimally invasive technique is a promising alternative for patients suffering from SVCAD, thus, avoiding median sternotomy and minithoracotomy.

Some studies for the assessment and evaluation of robotically assisted performance of anastomoses exist [3, 7]. There was no difference noticed regarding the quality comparing them to conventionally performed anastomoses. One of the issues still open for discussion remains an intraoperative assessment of the performed anastomosis. Postoperative angiography, which is always related to an increased workload (increased costs, patient risk and patient referral) is currently the only possibility for a reliable patency evaluation regarding the anastomosis. An interesting way to avoid these problems may be found in ultrasound [11].

The surgical procedure performed without any thoracotomy via a four point stab incision allows the integrity of the chest wall to be fully preserved. Postoperative convalescence is excellent with only small scars being visible [9].

The described surgical technique reflects a major step forward towards a *future* totally endoscopic surgical treatment of patients with more complex coronary artery pathology, especially for patients showing serious risk factors for extracorporal circulation and sternotomy related complications.

From the point of indication for operation, prospective studies will have to be performed in the future in order to verify the advantage of myocardial revascularization of single vessel coronary artery disease as compared to interventional therapy (PTCA/stent). Hereby, it is necessary to develop an interdisciplinary approach to meet the high demands necessary.

Summary

In the thrive towards a minimization of access in minimally invasive cardiac surgery (MICS), wrist-enhanced robotic instrumentation is currently leading to a turning point in the history of MICS as totally endoscopic coronary artery bypass (TECAB) grafting procedures become feasible. TECAB – using an endoscopic robotic surgical tool performing coronary artery bypass operations without any thoracotomy – reflects a major step towards a future endoscopic surgical treatment of patients with coronary artery disease (CAD). New technical innovations, such as the introduction of endoscopic stabilizers enables TECAB procedures of CAD via four 1-cm chest incisions on the beating heart and the avoidance of extracorporeal circulation. The currently applied standard at our institution for a endoscopic bypass procedure on the beating heart is presented.

References

1. Carpentier A, Loulmet D, Aupecle B, Berribi A, Relland (1999) Computerassisted cardiac surgery. The Lancet 353:379–380
2. Diegeler A, Thiele H, Falk V et al (2002) Comparison of stenting with minimally invasive bypass surgery for stenosis of the left anterior descending coronary artery. N Engl J Med 347: 561–566
3. Diodato LH, Scarborough JE, Domkowski PW et al (2002) Robotically assisted versus conventional freehand technique during beating heart anastomoses of the left internal thracic artery to left anterior descending artery. Ann Thorac Surg 73(3):852–859
4. Falk V, Diegeler A, Walther T, Bannusch J, Autschbach R, Mohr FW (2000) Total endoscopic coronary artery bypass grafting. Eur J Cardiothorac Surg 17(1):38–45
5. Falk V, Diegeler A, Walther T, Jacobs S, Raumans J, Mohr FW (2000) Total endoscopic off pump coronary artery bypass grafting. Heart Surg Forum 17(1):38–45
6. Falk V, Diegeler A, Walther T, Löscher N, Vogel B, Ulmann C, Rauch T, Mohr FW (1999) Endoscopic coronary artery bypass grafting on the beating heart using computer enhanced telemanipulation system. Heart Surg Forum 2(3):199–205
7. Falk V, Gummert J, Walther T, Hayesi M, Berry GJ, Mohr FW (1999) Quality of computer enhanced endoscopic coronary artery bypass graft anastomosis – comparison to conventional technique. Eur J Cardiothoracic Surg 13:260–266
8. Goy JJ, Eeckhout E, Burnand B, et al (1994) Coronary angioplasty versus left internal mammary artery grafting for isolated proximal left anterior descending artery stenosis. Lancet 343:1449
9. Kappert U, Cichon R, Schneider J et al (2001) Technique of closed chest coronary artery surgery on the beating heart. Eur J Cardiothorac Surg 20(4):765–769
10. Kappert U, Schneider J, Cichon R et al (2001) The development of robotic enhanced endoscopic surgery for the treatment of coronary artery disease. Circulation 104(Suppl. I):I-102–107
11. Klein P, Meijer R, Eikelaar JH, Gründeman PF, Borst C (2002) Epicardial ultrasound in off pump coronary artery bypass grafting: potential aid in intraoperative coronary diagnostic. Ann Thorac Surg 73(3):809–812

12. Loulmet D, Carpentier A, d'Attelis N et al (1999) First endoscopic coronary artery bypass grafting using computer assisted instruments. J Thorac Cardiovasc Surg 118:4–10
13. Mack MJ, Acuff TE, Casimir-Ahn H et al (1997) Video assisted coronary bypass grafting on the beating heart. Ann Thorac Surg 63 (6 Suppl):S100–103
14. Mohr FW, Falk, Diegeler A, Autschbach R (1999) Computer enhanced coronary artery bypass surgery. J Thorac Cardiovasc Surg 117:1212–1213
15. Reichenspurner H, Boehm DH, Gulbins H, Detter C, Damiano R, Mack M, Reichart B (1999) Robotically assisted endoscopic coronary artery bypass procedures without cardiopulmonary bypass. J Thorac Cardiovasc Surg 118:960–961
16. RITA Trial Participants (1993) Coronary angioplasty versus coronary artery bypass surgery: the Randomized Intervention Treatment of Angina (RITA) trial. Lancet 341:573
17. Shennib H, Bastawisy A, Mack MJ, Moll FH (1998) Computer assisted telemanipulation: an enabling technology for endoscopic coronary artery bypass. Ann Thorac Surg 66(3):1060–1063
18. Shennib H, Bastawisy A, McLoughlin J, Moll F (1999) Robotic enhanced telemanipulation enhances coronary artery bypass. J Thorac Cardiovasc Surg 117:310–313

CHAPTER 4 Minimally invasive conduit harvesting

Minimally invasive vein harvesting

I. Schade, B. Löwe

Introduction and history

In cardiac surgery, different bypass grafts are used, such as arterial grafts (mammary artery, radial artery, inferior epigastric artery and the right gastroepiploic artery) and venous grafts (great saphenous vein). Since 1968, venous bypass grafting has been a standard procedure for coronary revascularization in heart surgery. The use of the great saphenous vein was introduced by Favaloro [6].

The incision for harvesting of the great saphenous vein is the longest incision performed on the human body during surgery [4]. Traditionally, the vein was harvested on the medial side of the thigh and lower leg with a long incision from the ankle to the groin. The consequences were large wounds, related to bleeding, hematoma or infections. The graft harvested could be used as an aorto-coronary venous bypass [1].

During further development of surgical techniques, surgeons tried to reduce surgical trauma and at the same time improve cosmetic result. As in other surgical disciplines, minimally invasive techniques were introduced for routine use in heart surgery. What was expected from the new techniques compared to the standard procedure, was as a primary goal decrease of morbidity or mortality, while maintaining the quality of the procedure. Whether this is also true for vein harvesting remains to be clarified. In case of minimally invasive vein harvesting techniques, the primary goal should be a distinct decrease in complications.

Different harvesting techniques were developed for harvesting of the great saphenous vein, such as 1) the bridging technique, 2) video-assisted vein harvesting, and 3) endoscopic vein harvesting, in addition to the open technique.

This chapter in particularly discuses complications and cosmetic result of the bridging technique. The other two MIC techniques, which were mentioned above, will be discussed separately in the following chapters.

The bridging technique

To prepare for vein harvesting, the leg region is disinfected and covered with sterile drapes. The preferred leg for harvesting is rotated slightly outwards.

With the bridging technique, the great saphenous vein is harvested via several incisions of approx. 4 to 5 cm in length with bridges of skin in between. The first incision is made just above the medial malleolus and the vein is exposed in the fascia canal. In the area of the open incisions, harvesting is performed using a conventional technique with direct visibility. A small pair of scissors is used during preparation to dissect the vein from the fascia. It is essential to avoid direct lesions of the adventitia or the tributaries.

The segments of the vein harvested are cannulated with a bulb-headed cannula. The tributaries are closed proximally and distally using Ligaclips.

In the area of the skin bridges, the preparation of the vein is mainly performed under direct vision. The layers of skin and subcutaneous tissue above the vein are retracted using a Langenbeck's hook. The anterior and inferior preparation of the vein is partially performed with the pair of scissors and partially bluntly by finger. The tributaries are ligated intra-cavitally with a clip applicator and cut sharply. Depending on the training and manual skill of the surgeon, 6–8 cm of the vein can be harvested in this manner, until the next incision is made. In order to avoid too many incisions, the next incision is not made immediately at the end of the exposed section of the vein, but at a further 3–4 cm more distally. The preparation performed from the next incision can therefore be achieved in the proximal and distal direction, whereas the technique is entirely the same. During the learning phase, additional assisting incisions may be necessary to manage tributaries and to avoid unnecessary shearing forces at the vein. After the preparation is completed, the vein is closed in the thigh area with a 2/0 polyfile, not resorbable suture.

After careful hemostasis, the subcutaneous closure of the wound is performed using a 2/0 polyfile, not resorbable suture single or continuous suture technique. To avoid bleeding into the wound canal, Redon drains can be left in place but are not obligatory. To reduce the wound cavity after the skin is closed, a light elastic compression bandage is applied for about 48 hours. In patients with peripheral arterial occlusive disease, only a loose bandage is applied and the perfusion of the leg is monitored at regular intervals.

Using the procedure described above, vein harvesting over the entire length of the great saphenous vein is possible (Fig. 1).

A comparison of the bridging technique and conventional vein harvesting

The study of different vein harvesting techniques which was performed at our clinic showed significant differences intra-operatively as well as post-operatively. In approx. 50% of the veins which were harvested using the bridging technique the veins were removed from the thigh as well as the lower leg.

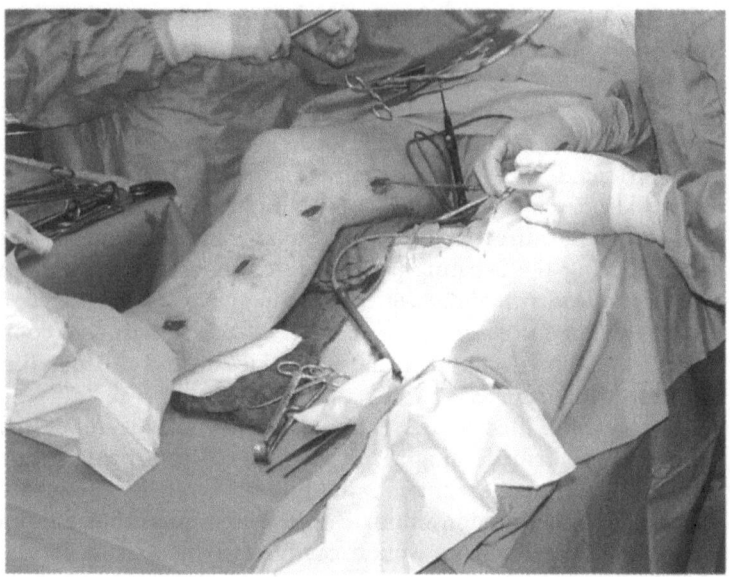

Fig. 1. Intra-operative representation of the bridging technique

Due to the significant (p < 0.05) faster closing time for the MIC technique, total time of vein harvesting including scin-suture is equally long for both groups. The operative blood loss, was also significantly lower (p < 0.000) in the MIC group (47.0 ± 47.4 ml) compared to the conventional group (178.0 ± 123.8 ml). In the group with the conventional procedure (n = 18 patients) twice as many Redon drains were used compared to the bridging technique (n = 9 patients; p < 0.05).

In the early post-operative phase, occurrence of hematoma, wound dehiscence and necrosis were used as a measure of trau-matization of the tissue. Thus, the occurrence of hematoma in 32 patients (64% of the total group) in the group where the conventional procedure was used was significantly higher (p < 0,05) compared to 10 patients (19.6%) in the bridging tech-nique group. Wound dehiscence was observed on the second

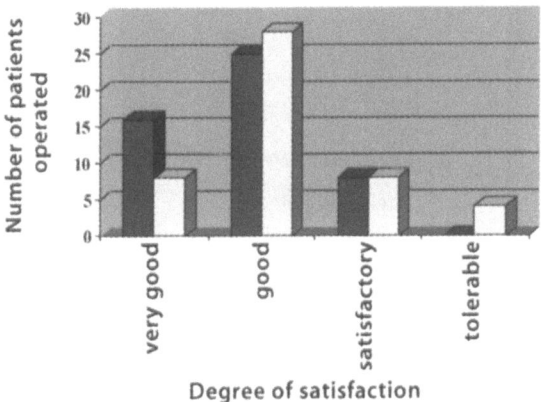

Fig. 2. Cosmetic satisfaction in the early post-operative phase (two weeks post-operatively; $p < 0.02$, shaded bars = bridging technique, open bars = conventional technique)

post-operative day in 6 patients (12%) in the conventional group compared to 2 patients (4%) in the bridging technique group. However these complications were no longer demonstrated on the fifth day after the operation in the latter group. Wound infections at a later point in time only occurred in the group with conventional operations. At no point in time were the subjective perceptions, such as wound pain, different for the two techniques.

Two weeks post-operatively, primary wound healing was significantly higher ($p < 0.05$) in the group where the minimally invasive technique was used. Secondary wound healing was observed frequently in the conventional vein harvesting group. Even at later post-operative points in time, the MIC group (bridging technique) had better results for subjective perceptions, such as pain ($p < 0.03$). Perception disorders ($p < 0.077$) and the cosmetic result ($p < 0.02$) were also better for the MIC group (Figs. 2 and 3).

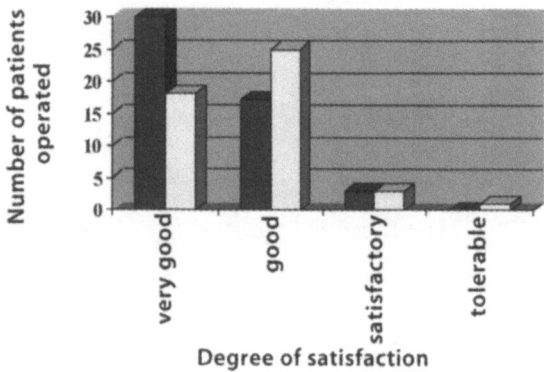

Fig. 3. Cosmetic satisfaction in the late post-operative phase (twelve weeks post-operatively; $p < 0.01$, shaded bars = bridging technique, open bars = conventional technique)

Summary

Today, vein harvesting for use in coronary artery bypass surgery can be performed using the conventional method with a long incision or the minimally invasive method using the bridging technique. With the use of minimally invasive procedures, the formation of large skin flaps extended, bleeding and long exposure to the environment can be avoided [14].

In contrast to the technique using the Mayo stripper [9, 10], the procedure using the bridging technique is performed under visibility. The preparation could be performed using a pair of scissors and did not have to be blunt. Depending on the degree of experience of the surgeon, the bridging technique is not too difficult even in obese patient and did not show a higher percentage of complications. In addition, it is possible at any time to switch from the minimally invasive to the conventional technique, while conversion rates of less than 5% are reported [11].

The literature provides only little information on practical use with regard to wound healing complications [5]. Most studies on this subject were performed on the conventional technique. Complications discussed were those mainly occurring in the case of large wound healing defects and prolonged surgical treatment [5]. The studies showed that a significantly higher morbidity is almost impossible [12, 14], whereas wound healing disturbances could still be observed [2, 3, 8, 13].

MELDRUM-HANNA et al. [9] described a wound complication rate of 0.9% in patients where the minimally invasive bridging technique was performed and which had better cosmetic results. Switching over to skin bridges with incisions resulted in significantly better wound healing with a reduction in wound healing complications from 21.7 to 8.8% [16]. Studies were able to show that compared with the conventional technique the use of the bridging technique allows a saphenectomy [15] with less wound pain and a lower infection rate.

An additional advantage of the described technique is the possibility of using conventional instruments, which makes the technique commercially attractive. TRAN et al. [15] evan demonstrated that vein harvesting using the bridging technique provides better results with regard to maintaining the endothelial structure than conventionally harvested veins. This is exceedingly essential to ensure that bypass function is not limited.

If at our institution segments of the great saphenous vein are harvested without using the endoscopical technique, e.g., due to either lack of experience on behalf of the surgeon or lack of endoscopic instruments, the saphenectomy is always performed using the bridging technique. The open conventional technique has been completely abandoned.

References

1. Allen KB, Shaar CD (1997) Endoscopic saphenous vein harvesting: minimally invasive video-assisted saphenectomy. Ann Thorac Surg 64:1183–1185
2. Allen KB, Griffith GL, Heimansohn DA, Robison RJ, Matheny RG et al (1998) Endoscopic versus traditional saphenous vein harvesting: a prospective, randomized trail. Ann Thorac Surg 66:26–32

3. Carpino PA, Khabbaz KR, Bojar RM, Rastegar H, Warner KG et al (2000) Clinical benefits of endoscopic vein harvesting in patients with risk factors for saphenectomy wound infections undergoing coronary artery bypass grafting. J Thorac Cardiovasc Surg 119:69–76

4. Cusimano RJ, Dale L, Butanny JW (1996) Minimally invasive cardiac surgery for removal of the greater saphenous vein. Can J Surg 39:386–388

5. DeLaria GA, Hunter JA, Goldin MD et al (1981) Leg wound complications associated with coronary revascularization. J Thorac Cardiovasc Surg 81:403–407

6. Favaloro RG (1968) Saphenous vein autograft replacement of severe segmental coronary artery occlusion: operative technique. Ann Thorac Surg 5:334–339

7. Lavee J, Schneiderman J, Yorav S, Shewach-Millet M, Adar R (1989) Complications of saphenous vein harvesting following coronary artery bypass surgery. J Cardiovasc Surg 30:989–991

8. Meldrum-Hanna W, Ross D, Johnson D et al (1986) An improved technique for long saphenous vein harvesting for coronary revascularization. Ann Thorac Surg 42:90–92

9. Meldrum-Hanna W, Ross D, Johnson D, Deal C (1986) Long saphenous vein harvesting. Aust N Z J Surg 81:403–407

10. Newman RV, Lammle G (1999) Minimally invasive vein harvest: new techniques with old tools. Ann Thorac Surg 67:571–572

11. Sellick JA Jr, Stelmach M, Mylotte JM (1991) Surveillance of surgical wound infections following open heart surgery. Infect Control Hosp Epidem 12:591–596

12. Slaughter MS, Gerchar DC, Pappas PS (1998) Modified minimally invasive technique for greater saphenous vein harvesting. Ann Thorac Surg 65:571–572

13. Tevaearai HT, Mueller XM, von Segesser LK (1997) Minimally invasive harvest of saphenous vein for coronary artery bypass grafting. Ann Thorac Surg 63:119–121

14. Tran HM, Paterson HS, Meldrum-Hanna W, Chard RB (1998) Tunneling versus open harvest technique in obtaining venous conduits for coronary bypass surgery. Eur J Cardiothorac Surg 14:602–606

15. Weiss VJ, Lin P, Lumsden AB (1999) Endoscopic vein harvest techniques for coronary and infrainguinal bypass. Semin Laparosc Surg 6:127–134

Minimally invasive vein harvesting – video-assisted vein harvesting

R. Coppoolse, W. Rees, M. G. Muniputanna, D. Oefler, H. Warnecke

Introduction

Minimally invasive vein harvesting by endoscopic techniques has become technically feasible during recent years. A variety of techniques have been developed in order to obviate long skin incisions (1–4, 6, 7, 9, 10, 13–15). These procedures, however, have raised limited enthusiasm and have not gained widespread acceptance. This is in contrast to the large scale scientific effort towards minimizing thoracic incisions. Saphenectomy, however, leads to far longer skin incisions and a much higher prevalence of wound complications and pain than median sternotomy. Although severe morbidity like sepsis or amputation are encountered only in rare instances (11), major complications such as wound dehiscence, excessive drainage, lymphangitis and delayed wound healing are reported in up to 24% of patients resulting in severe patient discomfort and additional cost (8, 11, 16). In spite of this, the operative technique of saphenectomy has not been improved significantly since the advent of coronary revascularization. Interrupted skin incisions were the only technical proposal for reducing these complications but were not generally accepted. However, starting in 1996, minimally invasive vein harvesting has been described as an alternative procedure in a few centers.

Surgical technique

Standard saphenous vein harvesting was performed by one longitudinal uninterrupted skin incision. Vein side branches were closed by clips. Saphenectomy and skin closure were performed by senior residents only. Skin closure was by absorbable intracutaneous suture. Suction drainage was used liberally when harvesting the saphenous vein from the thigh. Great care was taken to appropriately compress the leg by bandaging for 24 hours postoperatively. Our technique for minimally invasive endoscopic saphenectomy is performed with a commercially available endoscopic system (Karl Storz Endoskope, Tuttlingen, Germany) (Fig. 1). The system can be sterilized completely. No disposables are used.

Saphenectomy and median sternotomy with preparation of the left internal mammary artery are performed simultaneously. After disinfection, the leg is draped with an incision foil. A longitudinal incision of 3–4 cm length is performed at the medial aspect of the thigh, 5 to 10 cm above the knee. We found longitudinal incisions to be superior to transverse incisions, be-

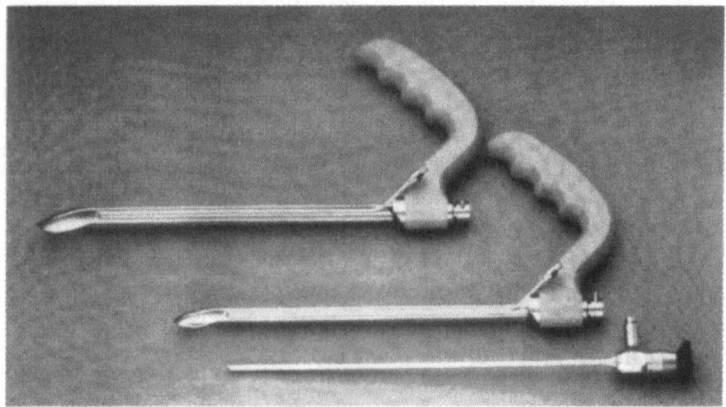

Fig. 1. Endoscopic system

cause preparation of the first centimeter of the vein is facilitated. After identification of the greater saphenous vein, the subcutaneous tunnel dissector carrying an endoscope is inserted. Surgery is performed under videoscopic view by a standard monitor. The essentials of our technique are as follows.

- The subcutaneous tunnel above the saphenous vein is created only by sharp dissection.
- No blunt dissection is allowed.
- Likewise, it is actively discouraged to use the tunnel dissector, which was originally designed for blunt tunnelling, in this manner. Uncontrolled bleeding and major shear forces on the vein graft may result.
- All major side branches are closed by clips.
- Bipolar cautery is appropriate for small side branches. The cauterization of large side branches is avoided as uncontrolled heat transfer towards the vein graft might result (Fig. 2).
- The use of the ring stripper instrument provided by the manufacturer is discouraged as side branches might be disrupted.

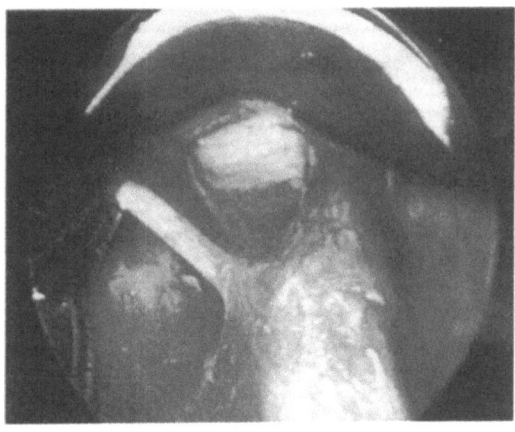

Fig. 2. Endoscopic view of the vein with side branch

The dissection process is carried forward up to the saphenous-femoral junction. A second incision of 3–4 cm length may be used proximally. Alternatively, an "Endoloop" ligature (Ethicon, Norderstedt, Germany) may be applied over the distal free end of the vein and advanced endoscopically to the groin. The saphenous vein is ligated proximally either by an "Endoloop" ligature, by clip or by direct visualized ligation via an incision in the groin.

During the learning curve, we especially recommend the use of additional incisions during the course of the vein, if difficulties are encountered in identifying side branches. These incisions may be directed at the tip of the tunnel dissector instrument and, thus, can be very short. During the introductory phase, a compromising strategy can be established, which allows for additional skin incisions in case of time restraints, bleeding or obscured vision (Fig. 3).

When additional vein length is required, the tunnel can be brought down to below the knee and the vein can be divided

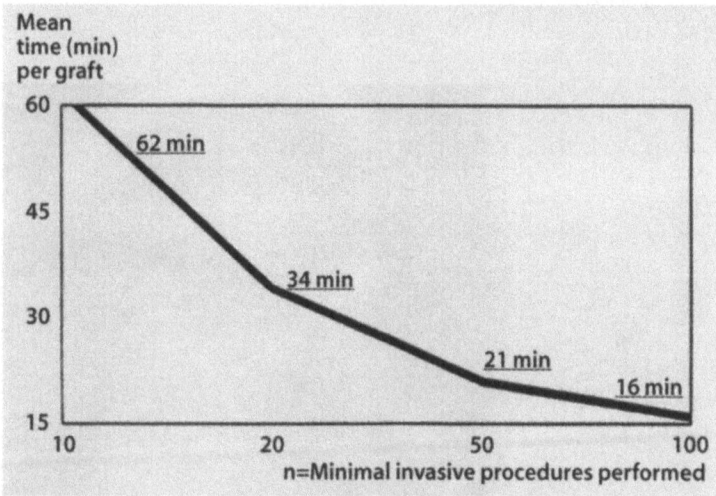

Fig. 3. Time per graft harvested in dependence of procedures performed

here, again either by "Endoloop" or direct ligature via an additional incision. Saphenectomy of the calf is technically more difficult due to the lack of subcutaneous tissue and is not recommended as a routine procedure.

Suction drainage of the tunnel is used liberally, but we do not find it essential. The leg is wrapped immediately after skin closure with elastic bandages in order to prevent hematoma, while the patient is fully heparinized on extracorporeal circulation.

Outcome

A prospective, randomized study investigated the method and outcome of minimal invasive harvested grafts showing following results in 300 patients each (5).

The introduction of endoscopic saphenectomy into a routine program was achieved with increasing training status of surgical senior residents and better familiarity with the procedure, leading to an increased acceptance of procedure.

Overall operation time did not differ significantly between both procedures (151 = 27 min for endoscopic saphenectomy vs. 145 = 31 min for conventional saphenectomy). Harvesting time per graft is shown in Fig. 3. An average of 2.17 vein grafts were used in patients with endoscopic harvesting vs. 2.2 grafts in conventional procedures. On average, 0.9 arterial grafts were additionally used resulting in a revascularization rate of 3.1 grafts per patient for both groups. Conversion from endoscopic to conventional saphenectomy was necessary in 1.6% of the patients. In 18 patients, a multitude of side branches leading to a difficult and time-consuming harvesting procedure made this necessary. In 5 patients conversion was necessary because of superficial course or varicose abnormalities of the saphenous vein.

Wound healing disturbances were encountered significantly more often in the conventional saphenectomy group. The results of the subgroup comparison of 300 patients with endo-

Table 1. Wound complications

	Comparative study	
	Minimally invasive n = 300	Conventional n = 300
Moderate ▌ Hematoma, superficial infection	5 (1.7%)	24 (8%)
Severe ▌ Surgical intervention required	0 (0%)	9 (3%)

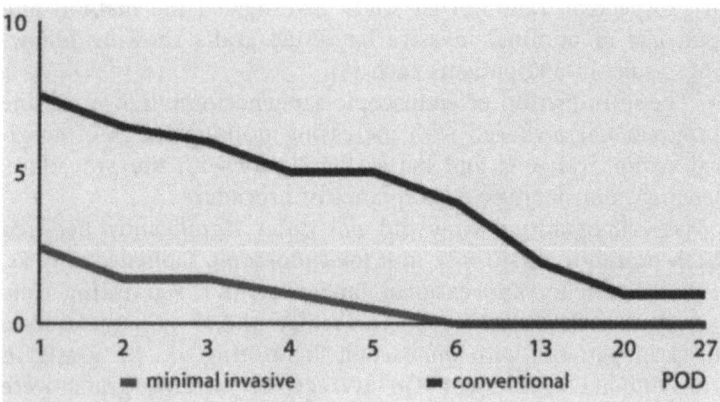

Fig. 4. Patients were asked to classify their pain on a slide ruler scale, graded from 0 (no pain) to 10 (unbearable pain) (17)

scopic saphenectomy compared to 300 patients concurrently operated on by conventional saphenectomy are given in Table 1. In these two groups, patient demographic data were comparable with regard to age (mean 71 years in the endoscopic group vs. mean 69 years), sex (187 vs. 173 male patients), body weight (79.4 vs. 77.3 kg) and prevalence of insulin-dependent diabetes.

Table 2. Postop clinical outcome: perioperative myocardial infarction

	Minimally invasive vein harvest	Conventional vein harvest
▌ CKMB > 10% CK	5 (1.66%)	7 (2.33%)
▌ Q-wave MI	3 (1%)	4 (1.33%)
▌ New wall hypokinesia	2 (0.66%)	3 (1%)

Table 3. Long-term results: mortality

Postoperative interval	Minimally invasive	Conventional
30 days	n = 4 (1.3%)	n = 5 (1.7%)
1 year	n = 8 (2,7%)	n = 11 (3.7%)
2 years	n = 15 (5%)	n = 16 (5.3%)
3 years	n = 18 (6%)	n = 20 (6.6%)

The perception of pain was more severe in patients after conventional saphenectomy. The pain for both groups during the first four postoperative weeks is illustrated in Fig. 4. Consequently postoperative mobilization was facilitated and patient discomfort reduced.

Histologic investigations showed no significant differences by means of stained light microscopy. There was no significant difference in early graft failure in either group. The diagnosis of peri-operative myocardial infarction was made in 1.9% of patients after endoscopic saphenectomy and 2.3% patients after conventional saphenectomy (Table 2).

No significant clinical outcome regarding postoperative myocardial infarction could be shown, as well as there was no change in midterm survival up to 3 years (Table 3).

Summary

Minimally invasive endoscopic vein harvesting can be performed as a routine procedure. Judged by the unchanged incidence of peri-operative myocardial infarctions and long-term results, graft quality appears to be unimpaired. The harvesting procedure can be incorporated into the operative time schedule without unduly lengthening operating room time. A higher level of surgical training and expertise is required, but this is by far outweighed by a reduced incidence of wound infection, less postoperative pain and a much superior cosmetic result.

References

1. Allen K, Griffith G, Heimansohn D, Robison R, Matheny R, Schier J, Fitzgerald E, Shaar C (1998) Endoscopic versus traditional saphenous vein harvesting: a prospective, randomised trial. Ann Thorac Surg 66:26–32
2. Black EA, Guzik TJ, West NE, Campbell K, Pillai R, Ratnatunga C, Channon KM (2001) Minimally invasive saphenous vein harvesting: effects on endothelial and smooth muscle function. Ann Thorac Surg 71(5):1503–1507
3. Cable D, Dearani J, Pfeifer E, Daly R, Schaff H (1998) Minimally invasive saphenous vein harvesting: endothelial integrity and early clinic results. Ann Thorac Surg 66:139–143
4. Cisowski M, Wites M, Gerber W, Drzewiecka-Gerber A, Bochenek A (2000) Minimally invasive saphenous vein harvesting for coronary artery bypass grafting – comparison of three less invasive methods. Med Sci Monit 6(4):735–739
5. Coppoolse R, Rees W, Krech R, Hufnagel M, Seufert K, Warnecke H (1999) Routine minimal invasive vein harvesting reduces postoperative morbidity in cardiac bypass procedures. Clinical report of 1400 patients. European Journal of Cardio-Thoracic Surgery 16(Suppl 2):S61–S66
6. Cusimano R, Dale L, Butany J (1996) Minimally invasive cardiac surgery for removal of the greater saphenous vein. Can J Surg 39(5):386–388

7. Davis Z, Jacobs H, Zhang M, Thomas C, Castellanos Y (1998) Endoscopic vein harvest for coronary artery bypass grafting: technique and outcomes. J Thorac Cardiovasc Surg 116:228–235
8. DeLaria G, Hunter J, Goldin M, Serry C, Javid H, Najafi H (1981) Leg wound complications with coronary revascularization. J Thorac Cardiovasc Surg 81:403–407
9. Dusterhoft V, Bauer M, Buz S, Schaumann B, Hetzer R (2001) Wound-healing disturbances after vein harvesting for CABG: a randomized trial to compare the minimally invasive direct vision and traditional approaches. Ann Thorac Surg 72(6):2038–2043
10. Fabricius AM, Diegeler A, Doll N, Weidenbach H, Mohr FW (2000) Minimally invasive saphenous vein harvesting techniques: morphology and postoperative outcome. Ann Thorac Surg 70(2): 473–478
11. Lee KS, Reinstein L (1986) Lower limb amputation of the donor site extremity after coronary artery bypass graft surgery. Arch Phys Med Rehabil 67:564–565
12. Lui WHD, Aitkenhead AR (1991) Comparison of contemporaneous and retrospective assessment of postoperatie pain using the visual analog scale. Br J Anaesth 67:768–771
13. Lumsden A, Eaves F, Ofenloch J, Jordan W (1996) Subcutaneous video-assisted saphenous vein harvest: report of the first 30 cases. Cardiovasc Surg 4(6):771–776
14. Reichenspurner H, Boehm D, Welz A, Reichart B (1998) Minimally invasive cardiac surgery – a fashion or an accepted surgical concept? Z Kardiol 87:594–603
15. Tevaearai H, Mueller X, von Segesser L (1997) Minimally invasive harvest of the saphenous vein for coronary artery bypass grafting. Ann Thorac Surg 63(6):119–121
16. Utley J, Thomason M, Wallce D (1989) Preoperative correlates of impaired wound healing after saphenous vein excision. J Thorac Surg 30:147–149
17. Lui WHD, Aitkenhead AR (1991)) Comparison of contampeianuous and retrospective assessment of postoperative pain using the visual analog scale. Br J Anaesth 67:768–771

Minimally invasive video-assisted endoscopic vein harvesting

A. Kapsalis, K. Alexiou

Introduction

Each year, surgery is performed in Germany on approx. 75000 patients with coronary artery disease (approx. 75% of all heart surgery). The material used for bypass surgery is arterial grafts and predominantly autologous veins, mainly the great saphenous vein which is taken in approximaly 95% of aorto-coronary bypass operations [4]. For conventional vein harvesting, the skin incision often runs along the entire length of have leg. Therefore, this skin incision is the longest incision made during any kind of surgical intervention on the human body. For several years, surgeons have tried to reduce the length of the skin incision applying different surgical techniques. They did not only have aesthetic aspects in mind: wound complications after saphenectomy are by no means rare in cardiac surgery [9]. The spectrum includes paresthesias, lymphatic edemas, hematomas, but also wound infections, skin necroses and in rare cases leg amputations [6, 9]. One of the minimally invasive techniques which has established itself beside the minimally invasive bridging technique is endoscopic video-assisted vein harvesting. It allows removal of the entire length of the great saphenous vein by a single incision of about 2 cm at the inside of the popliteal fossa. Beside the aesthetic benefit which is very important for the patient, a significant reduction in wound complications in the leg could be observed post-operatively [1, 2].

In addition to the minimally invasive bridging technique, endoscopic saphenectomy was established using the Guidant VasoView 4/5 EVH System in our clinic.

Pre-operative preparation

Evaluation of the great saphenous vein

Natural history

A prerequisite for using the great saphenous vein as a graft in aorto-coronary bypass surgery is good quality of the vein. If previously vein stripping, phlebosclerosation, trunk varicosis or a deep leg vein thrombosis is reported, the great saphenous vein should not be removed. Prior leg surgery or injuries should also be considered, especially if they occurred in the anatomical course of the great saphenous vein.

For patients with a superficial varicosis or varicosis of the tributaries, it is often the case that the trunk of the great saphenous vein is still of good quality and can thus be used for bypass grafting. In these cases, however, the surgeon should refrain from endoscopic vein harvesting because of the increased risk of injury to the vein or the varicose tributaries with subsequent bleeding causing limited visibility during preparation.

In patients with peripheral circulatory disturbances (peripheral arterial occlusive disease, diabetes mellitus, ulcus cruris), vein harvesting should be performed on the leg which is less affected. Endoscopic vein harvesting is even better in these cases compared to conventional saphenectomy. The risk of post-operative wound healing disturbances is significantly smaller because of less trauma [8].

Physical examination

For better evaluation of the leg veins, the patient should stand undressed in front of the examiner. The condition of the great saphenous vein which is well filled while the patient is standing can be properly evaluated with the fingers over the entire lower leg and the distal thigh.

By rhythmic tapping or smoothing down the distal great saphenous vein above the medial malleolus with the index finger of one hand, the other hand can feel from distal to proximal the pulsation which is caused synchronously with the palpation and showing the course of the great saphenous vein. It is important to identify the great saphenous vein in the knee area and mark the possible incision site with a waterproof pen. This will save valuable time intra-operatively during the preparation of the vein, particularly in very obese patients. Following this method, it is possible to already determine the course of the great saphenous veins and its tributaries the day before the operation and thus the more suitable leg for graft harvesting.

Phlebography

An x-ray examination using contrast for visualization of the leg vein system should only be performed, if a deep leg vein thrombosis is suspected. The phlebography should not be carried out immediately before bypass grafting. The highly osmolar contrast may cause endothelial damage to the intima of the veins.

▌ Preparation in the operating theater

Positioning of the patient

The patient is placed in the supine position. The legs are slightly bent by a knee support and rotated outward ("frog position"). The leg which is to be used for endoscopic vein harvesting should be lifted with an additional rolled piece of cloth in the knee area. This leads to an improvement in mobility for the long instruments, particularly during the preparation of the great saphenous vein.

Monitoring/instruments

We exclusively use the Guidant VasoView Uniport 4/5 EVH System for endoscopic vein harvesting. It includes a long endoscope with a conical tip and a built-in C-ring, a long bipolar pair of scissors as well as a port with a sealing balloon and a connector for CO_2 insufflation (Fig. 1). In addition, a 5 mm or 7 mm 0° optics, an extension cord for the bipolar pair of scissors, a light cable and an extension cord for the CO_2 insufflation device are required. These are connected to a tower unit with a monitor, camera, cold light source, CO_2 insufflator and diathermy device.

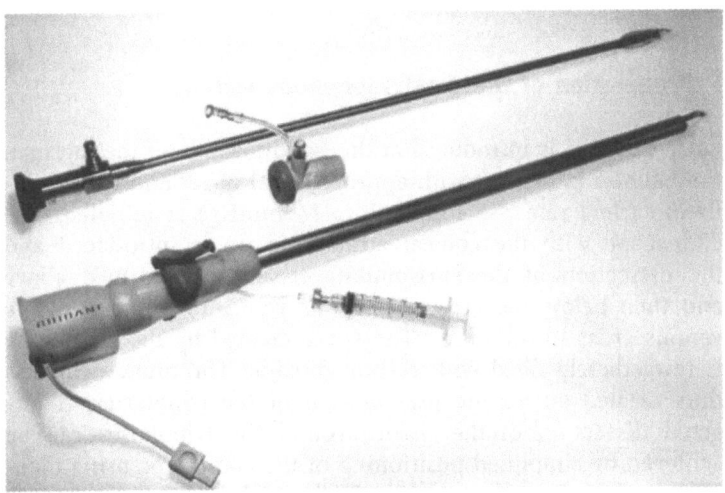

Fig. 1. The Guidant VasoView 5 EVH System with 7 mm endoscope

Surgical technique

Presentation of the great saphenous vein

A skin incision of 2 cm is performed directly above the great saphenous vein at the medial side of the knee in the longitudinal direction. It allows the preparation of the great saphenous vein along its entire length (lower leg and thigh) without an additional incision. Make sure that the incision is not longer than 2.5 cm, otherwise the preparation channel may not be sealed sufficiently to the outside after the port has been introduced and the balloon inflated.

By presenting and preparing the great saphenous vein with conventional instruments in the area of the incision as well as 3–4 cm proximal and distal to the skin incision, sufficient space is created for the introduction of the port. Possible tributaries in this area must be ligated and cut.

Preparation of the great saphenous vein

Once the port is introduced at the proximal side of the incision, the balloon is inflated with approx. 15 ml of air and CO_2 insufflation (flow rate 3–5 l/min, P_{max} 14 mmHg) is initiated. The endoscope with the conical atraumatic tip is introduced and the dissection of the surrounding tissue is performed above and then below the great saphenous vein into the area of the venous cross in the groin. The space created by the endoscope is immediately filled with carbon dioxide. The tunnel which is thus created allows the presentation of the tributaries. A targeted dissection of the tissue around the tributaries can be achieved by simplified positioning of the endoscope using manual pressure from the outside. At the end of the dissection all tributaries should be identified and exposed over a length of at least 3–4 mm. Subsequently, the port is removed and repositioned at the distal side of the incision in the direction of the lower leg. The preparation of the great saphenous vein of the lower leg is performed in the same way until just before the medial malleolus.

▌ Severing the tributaries

The conical tip is removed and the bipolar pair of scissors is introduced into the endoscope channel. Using the C-ring, the tributaries are visualized and positioned for dissection with the bipolar pair of scissors by simultaneous cutting and coagulating (Fig. 2). Large tributaries should be cut last, because side branch bleeding may limit visibility. In any case, the system includes a built-in flushing function. Through a small opening in the C-ring it is possible to spray saline onto the optics and clear away blood or fat particles without removing the endoscope. Tributaries should not be cut without sufficient exposure because of the risk of thermal vein injury. Further exposure and mobilization of these tributaries is possible by gently retracting them with the C-ring and simultaneous blunt and sharp dissection – fenestration – of the tissue around with the bipolar scissors. If sufficient exposure of the tributary is not achieved, an additional small skin incision above, allows direct visualization at the end of the preparation. Then the great saphenous vein is again loaded onto the C-ring and checked from distal to proximal over the entire length for remaining tributaries.

▌ Harvesting the great saphenous vein

A small clamp is introduced via a small stab incision (5 mm) in the groin and proximal to the medial malleolus, and under endoscopic visual control the great saphenous vein is grasped. With the bipolar pair of scissors the vein is then removed from the inside. Subsequently, the venous stump is pulled out, ligated and put back into place. Finally, the harvested vein is cannulated and flushed with heparinized saline. The tributaries are clipped and the vein is checked for sealing.

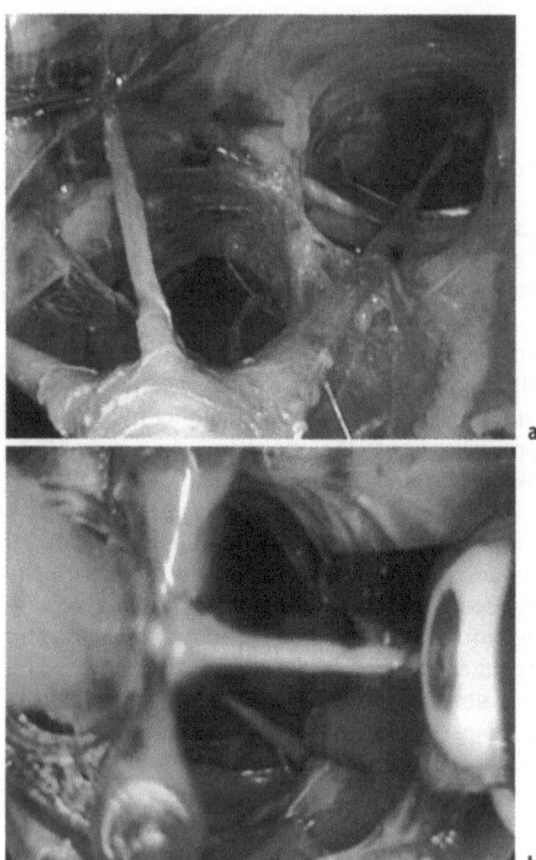

Fig. 2. a A full scope view. **b** Use of cradle and scissor to cut and coagulate the tributaries

Closure of wound

The wound at the knee is closed with subcutaneous and intra-cutaneous sutures. The adaptation of the edges of the small skin incisions is performed using Steri-Strips. Introduction of a

Redon drain is not obligatory. After a sterile dressing is applied, the leg is wrapped with elastic bandages.

Summary

The above endoscopic technique allows an easy, safe and fast endoscopic preparation of the great saphenous vein. Due to the conical atraumatic endoscope tip the dissection of vein from the surrounding tissue as well as the exposure of the tributaries is simplified. The continuous insufflation of carbon dioxide ensures a subcutaneous working channel with excellent visibility and the bipolar pair of scissors is a safe method to cut the tributaries. An experienced surgeon can handle the system well after a learning curve of 10–15 sessions [7]. In comparison to conventional vein harvesting the preparation time for the endoscopic technique is slightly longer, but the total time for also closing the leg wound is even less [3]. By selecting the incision at the medial side of the knee, the great saphenous vein can be either harvested from the lower leg or the thigh or both. With a total incision length of 3.0–3.5 cm a vein of up to 70 cm can be harvested (Fig. 3). Endoscopic vein harvesting from the thigh is easier than from the lower leg because of the anatomical situation (less and larger tributaries, no superficial veins). Therefore, the vein from the thigh should be preferred for preparation during the initial endoscopic sessions.

In summary our own experience shows that endoscopic vein harvesting is a superior alternative to the conventional methods, because of the reduction in wound healing complications, faster mobilization of the patients, reduction of the hospital stay, significant improvement of the cosmetic results, and reduced post-operative pain [1, 2, 5].

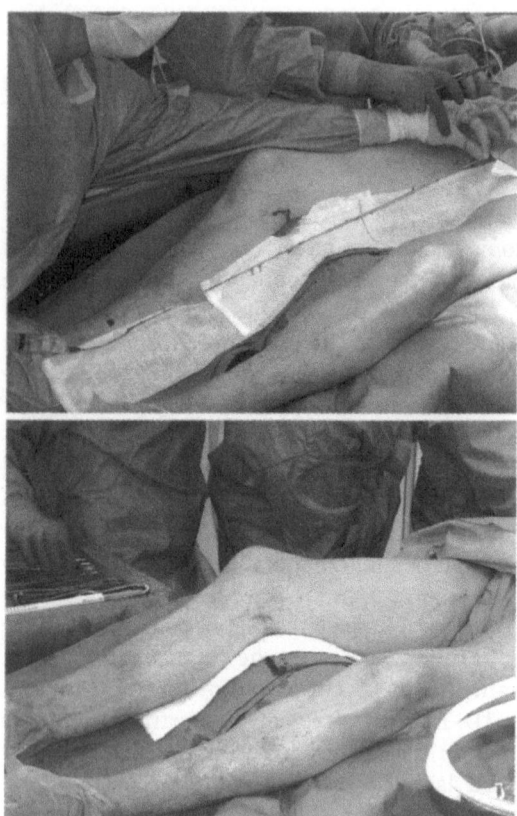

Fig. 3. A 70 cm vein harvested with a 2 cm incision at the medial side of knee and two small stab incisions (each 5 mm) in the groin and above the medial malleolus

References

1. Allen KB, Shaar CJ (1997) Endoscopic saphenous vein harvesting. Ann Thorac Surg 64:265–266
2. Cable DG, Dearani JA (1997) Endoscopic vein harvesting: minimally invasive video-assisted saphenectomy. Ann Thorac Surg 64:1183–1185
3. Davis Z, Jacobs HK, Zhang M, Thomas C, Castellanos Y (1998) Endoscopic vein harvest for coronary artery bypass grafting: technique and outcomes. J Thorac Cardiovasc Surg 116:228–235
4. Düsterhöft V, Bauer M, Zurbrügg HR, Sänger S, Bauer A, Buz S, Hetzer R (2000) Die traditionelle und die minimal-invasive Saphenektomie in der aortokoronaren Bypasschirurgie. Z Herz- Thorax-Gefäßchir 14:204–211
5. Jordan WD, Voellinger DC, Schroeder PT, McDowell HA (1997) Video-assisted saphenous vein harvest: the evolution of a new technique. J Vasc Surg 26:405–414
6. Lee KS, Reinstein L (1986) Lower limb amputation of the donor site extremity after coronary artery bypass graft surgery. Arch Phys Med Rehabil 67:564–565
7. Lumpsen AB, Eaves FF (1994) Focus on technique: subcutaneous, video-assisted saphenous vein harvest. Vasc surg 7:43–55
8. Lutz Ch, Schöllhorn J, Rump LC, Schwarzkopf G, Beyersdorf F (1999) Die Methode der minimalinvasiven, endoskopischen, video-assistierten Venenentnahme. Z Kardiol 88(Suppl 4):IV/35–IV/41
9. Wipke-Tevis DD, Stotts NA, Skov P, Carrieri-Kohlman V (1996) Frequency, manifestations, and correlates of impaired healing of saphenous vein harvest incisions. Heart Lung 25:108–116

Advances in minimally invasive harvesting of the radial artery for coronary bypass grafting

U. ROSENDAHL

Introduction

The radial artery, introduced by Carpentier in 1973 [4], abandoned shortly afterwards because of unsatisfactory early results, has enjoyed a revival since its re-introduction by Acar in 1992 due to unexpected long-term patency rates [1]. Because of these superior patency rates compared to venous grafts, the radial artery is used increasingly more for coronary bypass grafting [12].

It is important to notice that before this artery is taken into consideration as a conduit for coronary artery bypass grafting, non-invasive evaluation of the circulation of the hand usually the non-dominant, has to be applied. Different methods have been described by several authors [9, 11].

The brachioradial muscle covers the proximal part of the radial artery, distally it then emerges between this muscle and the flexor carpi radial muscle to lie superficially, only to be covered by the deep fascia, subcutaneous tissue and the skin [3, 10, 15]. The artery itself has approximately 17 perforating arteries, which have to be taken care off while harvesting it.

The traditional, open harvesting technique for the radial artery involves a 23–25 cm longitudinal incision from the wrist to the elbow and the dissection along the brachioradial muscle. Several important anatomic structures, like the superficial radial nerve, the lateral antebrachial cutaneous nerve, and the superficial palmar artery, have to be taken into consideration while dissecting the radial artery in the open fashion, in order to achieve an excellent postoperative result. But even with the most accurate surgical technique, the traditional, open harvesting technique is invariably associated with an high percentage of postoperative obstacles, like hematoma, pain at the harvesting site and loss of sensibility due to injury of sensitive nerves, impending patients quick and full recovery. Wound infections and extensive scaring often disable patients for a long time after conventional harvesting has been applied [5].

The first attempt to reduce the incidence of traumatic tissue injury resulted in the so-called "tunnel technique" or skip-incision approach. Since then, several minimally invasive methods for radial artery harvesting have been developed and are presently in use.

▊ "Tunnel technique or skip-incision technique"

Two or, depending on the length of the forearm, three about 3 cm long skin incisions are made along the forearm. The forearm is therefore divided in three parts and the incisions are made directly over the radial artery, allowing an easy approach to each of the thirds. Starting from the distal incision, a tunnel over the radial artery is dissected in a blunt and sharp way in both directions. Side branches are isolated and divided under direct vision as far as the incisions allow direct view [13]. This method allows for a "less invasive" approach, with reduced morbidity due to the harvesting maneuver, but due to the fact that an additional assistant is needed to maintain retraction during the harvesting process, it cannot regularly be applied in daily practice.

Minimally harvesting using a cold light armed retractor system

A minimally invasive harvesting technique which can be applied by any surgeon almost without the well-known "pitfalls" of a long ongoing "learning curve" is made possible by a rather simple retractor system. This method allows any surgeon to harvest the RA in a minimally invasive fashion after a short learning phase, with minimal technical equipment, in almost the same time as the conventional harvesting would take.

A cold light armed, retractor system (Genzyme Saphlite®) enables the surgeon to harvest the entire radial artery over a 3 cm longitudinal incision at the middle region of the forearm.

Technique

In order to harvest the radial artery, the proposed arm is positioned 45° out of the operating table. An approximately 3 cm longitudinal incision halfway down the underarm has to be performed along the belly of the brachio-radial muscle (Fig. 1).

The subcutaneous tissue and the fascia over the brachio-radial and the flexor carpi radial muscles are dissected, taking care of the lateral antebrachial cutaneous nerve (LABCN). The LABCN is an important nerve for the sensory enervation of the radial aspect of the volar forearm and parts of the dorsal aspect of the forearm and hand. Great care has to be taken in order to preserve it [6].

In the next step the so-called MW-3 (brachio-radial, extensor carpi radial longus and the extensor carpi radial brevis) muscles are laterally mobilized. Once these muscles have been lateralized, the radial artery with its concomitant veins is visualized and placed on a vessel loop.

From the medial forearm incision a tunnel over the superior aspect of the radial artery is established by blunt and partly

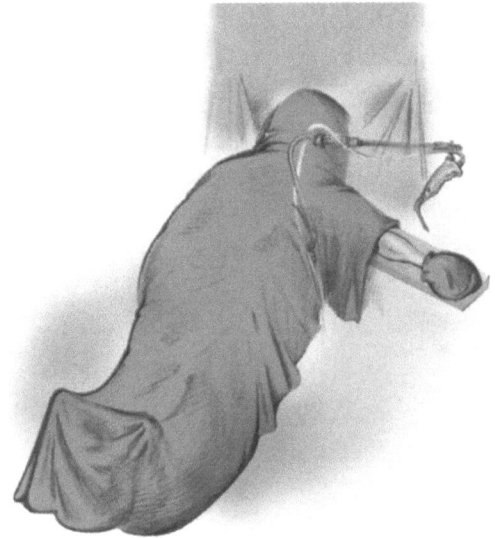

Fig. 1. Operative field

sharp dissection in a proximal and distal direction. The retractor with the fitted cold-light visualization system (Genzyme Corp. – GenzArm®, SaphLITE®) is introduced into the incision in the proximal direction, lifting the tissue over the superior aspect of the radial artery, thus, enabling visualization of the entire artery in the tunnel. The retractor-system can be positioned in any angle, a pneumatic systems allows a stable and quick fixation of the arm in the once chosen position.

The dissection proceeds with the preparation and ligation of all perforating branches using a vessel loop until the branching of the recurrent radial artery has been reached (Fig. 2).

At this point the proximal radial artery is divided and ligated using a 3/0 non-resorbable suture. Hemoclips are used in order to dissect the branches off the radial artery which, especially in very proximally or distally positioned perforating vessels, has proved to be very tedious and time consuming. A superior dissection-technique can be achieved through the use of a so-called ultrasonic-scalpel (Ethicon EndoSurgery®, Johnson &

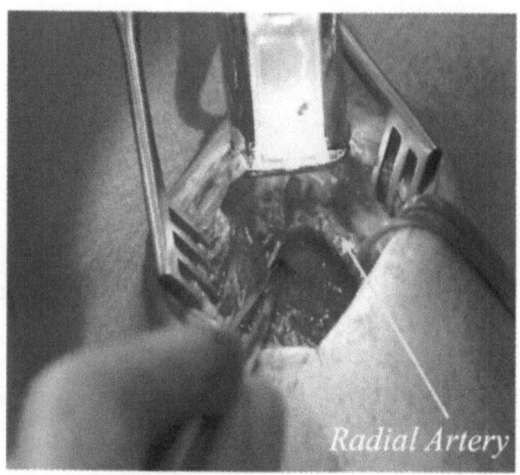

Radial Artery

Fig. 2. Retractor in incision

Johnson®), only larger branches are secured with hemoclips. Using this device, the minimally invasive harvesting technique can be accelerated enormously.

Dissection of the distal part of the radial artery is taken out 1–1.5 cm from the wrist, where it is ligated with a 3/0 non-resorbable suture and dissected. In order to facilitate distal ligation of the radial artery, an additional 1 cm skin incision might be needed distally in some cases where vision of the distal ligation site is not satisfying. This additional incision should be done in all cases where access to the distal part of the artery is somewhat awkward and proper ligation can not be done securely as bleeding from the distal stump of the artery might lead to unnecessary morbidity and ongoing complaints of the patient.

A wound drain has to be inserted only in cases where a mostly bloodless operating field cannot be obtained.

Wound closure is performed with a 3/0 resorbable suture subcutaneously and 4/0 resorbable suture intracutaneously. The forearm is then dressed with an elastic bandage for 48 hours. Afterwards no further bandaging is necessary.

After a short learning period, the average harvesting time for a radial artery graft is about 20–25 minutes. The average length of a graft harvested in this way is about 16–20 cm, usually enough to perform a total arterial revascularization in common coronary artery bypass grafting.

Comment

Possible spasm of the radial artery [7, 8] caused by this minimally invasive harvesting method have so far not been observed, as intra-operative transit-time Doppler flow measurement, which have been regularly performed in all cases, showed comparable excellent results. Three years results regarding performance of radial arteries, harvested in a minimally invasive fashion, did not differ from conventionally harvested radial arteries.

References

1. Acar C, Frage A, Chardigny C, Beyssen B, Pagny JY, Grare P, Fabiani JN, Deloche A, Guermonprez JL, Carpentier A (1993) Use of the radial artery for coronary artery bypass. A new experience after 20 years. Arch Mal Coeur Vaiss 86(12):1683–1689
2. Acar C, Ramsheyi A, Pagny JY, Jebara V, Barrier P, Fabiani JN, Deloche A, Guermonprez JL, Carpentier A (1998) The radial artery for coronary artery bypass grafting: clinical and angiographic results at five years. J Thorac Cardiovasc Surg 116(6):981–989
3. Buxton B, Fuller J, Geer J et al (1996) The radial artery as a bypass graft. Curr Opin Cardiol 11: 591–598 (review)
4. Carpentier A, Guermonprez JL, Deloche A, Frechette C, DuBost C (1973) The aorta-to-coronary radial artery bypass graft. A technique avoiding pathological changes in grafts. Ann Thorac Surg 16(2):111–121

5. Galajada Z, Péterffy Á (2001) Minimally invasive harvesting of the radial artery as a coronary artery bypass graft. Ann Thorac Surg 72:291–293

6. Greene MA, Malias MA (2001) Arm complications after radial artery procurement for coronary bypass operation. Ann Thorac Surg 72: 126–128

7. Gurevitch J, Miller HI, Shapira I, Kramer A, Paz Y, Matsa M, Mohr, R, Yakirevich V (1997) High-dose isosorbide dinitrate for myocardial revascularization with composite grafts. Ann Thorac Surg 63:382–387

8. He G-W, Yang C-Q (1996) Use of verapamil and nitrogycerin solution in preparation of radial artery for coronary grafting. Ann Thorac Surg 61:610–614

9. Jarvis MA, Jarvis Cl, Jones PR, Spyt TJ (2000) Reliability of Allen's test in selection of patients for radial artery harvest. Ann Thorac Sur 70(4):1362–1365

10. Ryes At, Frame R, Brodman RF (1995) Technique for harvesting the radial artery as a coronary artery bypass. Ann Thorac Surg 59(1):118–126

11. Starnes S, Wolk SW, Lampmann RM et al (1999) Non-invasive evaluation of hand circulation before radial artery harvest for coronary artery bypass grafting. J Thorac cardiovasc Surg 117:261–266

12. Tatoulis J, Buxton BF, Fuller JA, Royse AG (1999) Total arterial coronary revascularization: techniques and results in 3220 patients. Ann Thorac Surg 68:2093–2099

13. Terada Y, Uchida A, Fukuda I, Hochberg J, Mitsu T, Sato F (1998) Endoscopic harvesting of the radial artery as a coronary artery bypass graft. Ann Thorac Surg 66(6):2123–2124

14. Trick WE, Scheckler WE, Tkras JI, Jones KC, Smith EM, Reppen ML, Jarvis WR (2000) Risk factors for radial artery harvest site infection following coronary artery bypass graft surgery. Clin Infect Dis 30(2):270

15. Uchida, A, Hochberg J, Terada Y et al (1998) Endoscopic harvesting of radial artery grafts for coronary artery bypass. Ann Plast Surg 41:459–463

Endoscopic radial artery harvest

R. H. MILES, R. E. KOLLPAINTER

The history of the radial artery

The use of the radial artery as a conduit in coronary bypass surgery was first described by Carpentier et al., in 1973 [3]. This initial experience detailed 30 patients, in whom 40 radial arteries were utilized. Short-term results were encouraging with patency rates greater than 90% in grafts 1 to 10 months after implant. However, the radial artery was essentially abandoned when mid-term results (at 2 years) revealed that approximately one-third of the radial artery grafts displayed "severe generalized stenosis" [4, 5]. These results were attributed to traumatic harvesting techniques and the predilection of spasm in the radial artery [3, 5].

Eighteen years later, Acar et al., reported that some of these same radial artery grafts, previously demonstrated to be "occluded," were now without angiographic evidence of intimal disease or narrowing [1]. These findings prompted a re-evaluation of the radial artery as a conduit for bypass. In 1992, Acar et al. described their initial experience with 122 radial arteries in 104 patients [1]. They found graft patency to be 100% at 2 weeks, and greater than 93% at 1 year. The improved outcomes were attributed to more fastidious harvesting techniques, removal of the artery as a pedicled graft with the accompanying *venae comitantes* (rather than skeletonized), and use of peri-operative vasodilators [1].

Recently, Tatoulis et al. published their 5 year experience utilizing 8420 radial arteries for bypass in 6646 patients [10]. Follow-up angiography was performed in 369 patients, and 90.2% of the radial artery grafts were found to be patent. These findings have initiated a renewed interest in the radial artery as a conduit for bypass.

Preoperative evaluation

Standard evaluation of the forearm and hand circulation is initially performed by the modified Allen's test. Both the radial and ulnar arteries are compressed manually and several fist clenches are performed over 30 seconds to "exsanguinate" the hand. Ulnar artery compression is then released. Reperfusion of the entire hand within 5 seconds is considered excellent; within 10 seconds is considered acceptable; and greater than 10 seconds unacceptable. While some feel that this is adequate, we perform a more objective evaluation utilizing Doppler phlethysmography. By placing a pulse oximeter on the thumb when performing the Allen's test, one can assess oxygen saturation and waveform of isolated ulnar artery hand perfusion. If oxygen saturation and waveform return to baseline within 5 seconds, ulnar artery blood flow to the hand is sufficient to allow radial artery removal.

Contraindications to radial artery use may include an abnormal Allen's test, prior trauma or surgery to the relevant upper limb, known subclavian stenosis or brachial stenosis, need for hemodialysis, history of vasculitis, Raynaud's phenomenon, scleroderma, and radial artery calcification.

"Traditional" radial artery harvesting

The "traditional" method of open radial artery harvest requires a curvilinear incision on the volar surface of the forearm from the radial styloid process to the lateral aspect of the biceps tendon, just below the flexion crease of the elbow. The subcutaneous tissues are divided and the underlying brachioradialis muscle is retracted laterally. This exposes the lateral intermuscular fascia, which is then divided sharply to expose the radial artery pedicle.

Dissection of the radial artery and *venae comitantes* as a pedicle is then performed by dividing the radial artery side branches, which are numerous. The traditional method has been to clip the radial side of the tributary and divide the patient side with monopolar electrocautery [9]. Recently, the harmonic scalpel/shears have been utilized for more expedient division of side branches.

Endoscopic radial artery harvest

We have developed a technique that utilizes a standard extremity tourniquet. The tourniquet facilitates a bloodless field during the procedure, which is particularly beneficial during the learning curve. At the time of surgery, a tourniquet is placed high on the upper arm. The arm is then positioned on an arm board at a 90° angle prior to prepping and draping the patient. An intravenous nitroglycerin drip at 5 micrograms/kilogram/minute is initiated to attenuate radial artery spasm. The forearm is supinated and a 3 centimeter longitudinal incision is made between the flexor carpi radialis tendon and the radial styloid process, just proximal to the thenar eminence. This incision is chosen to minimize the risk of damage (or transection) to the lateral branch of the superficial radial nerve. Care is taken not to cross the wrist crease to avoid subsequent flexion difficulties.

Initial dissection is carried out to identify the radial artery and the *venae comitantes*. The lateral intermuscular fascia is sharply divided under direct vision. Once exposed, the forearm is wrapped tightly with a 4 inch Esmark^{TM} bandage (Medline, Mundelein, IL) to the elbow. The tourniquet is then inflated to 75 mmHg above the patients' systolic blood pressure (usually 200–250 mmHg) and the Esmark^{TM} wrap is then released. The forearm is supinated and extended, a rolled towel is placed under the wrist and the wrist is secured into place with an additional towel and towel clips.

▐ Endoscopic radial artery harvesting with the Guidant Uniport System

A 5 mm 0-degree fiberoptic endoscope (Guidant, Menlo Park, CA) is inserted into a conical tip dissection cannula (CDC) (Guidant, Menlo Park, CA) that is connected to a fiberoptic video system. The CDC is inserted into the incision and careful dissection posterior to the radial artery is performed to the elbow crease. The CDC is removed from the tunnel and the short port balloon tipped trochar (BTT) with a CDC seal (Guidant, Menlo Park, CA) is inserted into the incision. The balloon is inflated with 10 mL of air to seal the incision. Standard gas tubing is attached to the BTT port and CO_2 insufflation at 2 liters/minute (to a pressure of 10–15 mmHg) is utilized for tunnel expansion. The CDC is inserted through the BTT port and dissection of the radial artery is performed anteriorly. This is continued to the antecubital fossa by slipping the CDC under the lateral intermuscular fascia and lifting the tip anteriorly to put the dissection pressure against the fascia and not the radial artery. The end point of our dissection is either the identification of the recurrent radial artery branch or a large venous plexus that exists just proximal to the antecubital fossa. Lateral dissection is then performed. A "window" in the tissue is created laterally on both sides of the artery with the CDC every 1–2 centimeters down its entire length, avoiding direct contact with the artery itself. During the lateral dissection, side branches are identified but not dissected out.

After being connected to the fiberoptic scope, a Uniport Plus™ C-ring Dissector (Guidant, Menlo Park, CA) preloaded with 55 centimeter flexible scissors (Guidant, Menlo Park, CA) is then inserted through the BTT port. A fasciotomy of the lateral intermuscular septum the length of the forearm is then performed. Dividing the fascia increases the tunnel area and obviates the risk of compartment syndrome. Any anterior tributaries are divided with bipolar electrocautery. The tissue and tributaries are identified laterally on each side of the radial artery pedicle and are also divided with bipolar electrocautery. The C-ring of the dissector is utilized in standard fashion to aid in the division of posterior tributaries. "Running" the radial artery and accompanying *venae comitantes* with the C-ring confirms division of all side branches.

Endoscopic radial artery harvesting with the Ethicon Clearglide Endoscopic Vessel Harvesting System

The Ethicon Ultra-Retractor™ (Cardiovations, Somerville, NJ) is inserted into the incision and advanced 1–2 cm over the lateral intermuscular fascia. With the exposed harmonic shears blade pointed away from the radial artery, the section of fascia under the retractor is divided. The radial artery is rolled from side to side with the harmonic shears to identify the medial and lateral side branches. Once identified, the side branches are divided. The process is then repeated, at 1 cm intervals, down the length of the arm to the antecubital fossa. A vessel dissector is placed around the radial artery pedicle and is advanced along the length of the artery to locate and divide any missed posterior tributaries.

▮ Division of the radial artery and completion of the procedure

Division of the radial artery proximally is performed first. The endoscope is advanced to the end of the tunnel (at the elbow). Using trans-illumination, any superficial veins are identified and a stab incision is made with a # 11 blade into the tunnel. A mosquito clamp is inserted into the stab wound, and the radial artery and accompanying *venae comitantes* are grasped. The radial artery is divided *in situ* with endoscopic scissors, but without electrocautery. The radial artery stump is pulled through the stab incision and suture ligated. Alternatively, two separate snare loops with 2-0 monofilament suture can be utilized to ligate the artery proximally, thus, avoiding the stab incision. Division of the distal radial artery is carried out under direct vision through the wrist incision after distal artery suture ligation.

The wrist incision is then closed with 4-0 monofilament suture. The stab incision, when performed, is closed with Mastisol® and a Steri-Stip™. The forearm is wrapped with gauze and an elastic bandage. The tourniquet is then completely released. Capillary refill or pulse oximetry confirms ulnar patency. Postoperatively, the elastic wrap is removed within 4 hours of the operative procedure.

Once removed, the radial artery is *gently* flushed with heparinized saline and the side branches are ligated with hemoclips or 7-0 Prolene (when the branch is too short to clip). This step is obviously unnecessary when harmonic shears are utilized. The artery is then gently flushed with a blood and heparin solution to identify any missed branches, and is stored in a dilute papaverine solution until grafting is undertaken.

Discussion

It has been our desire to develop an endoscopic technique that would maximize equipment utilization, minimize cost, and facilitate routine harvest of the radial artery. The tourniquet technique for endoscopic radial artery harvest was initially reported by Uchida, et al., in 6 patients, but utilized equipment not readily available in most cardiac surgery operating suites [11]. Although the surgical skill required for endoscopic radial artery harvest is greater than that required for endoscopic vein harvest, we would suggest that either technique can be mastered with a short learning curve, provided one has obtained adequate comfort with endoscopic vein harvest.

The tourniquet technique

The tourniquet is utilized as a protective measure and can be used with either system. It is highly recommended with the Guidant system as bipolar electrocautery does not seal the radial artery tributaries. It may be less important with the Ethicon system and harmonics. With either approach, a conversion to open technique because of bleeding can be avoided with this simple, but effective, adjunct. Modern pneumatic tourniquets are designed to minimize the incidence of complications, and prospective randomized trials have found no adverse effects in extremity surgery when utilized properly [2, 7]. For surgical procedures of the upper extremity, the recommended tourniquet pressure should be 50–75 mmHg above the systolic arm blood pressure. It is also recommended that the widest cuff be placed as high up on the arm as possible. In general, tourniquet times are limited to a maximum of 2 hours for limb surgery. This recommendation has been based on functional, histologic, metabolic, and clinical studies [12]. Endoscopic harvesting of the radial artery with either technique can easily be completed in less than 1 hour. In our initial experience of 50 patients, our tourniquet time averaged 36.7 minutes.

█ Electrocautery vs. harmonics

Two technologies are currently being utilized in endoscopic radial artery dissection to facilitate side branch division: bipolar electrocautery and harmonics.

Bipolar electrocautery can be used safely if coagulation is performed at least 2 millimeters from the main vessel [6]. This protects against lateral thermal tissue injury and also minimizes radial artery spasm. Control of the electrocautery distance is easily maintained with the Guidant system throughout the length of the forearm, as it is an "in-line" system with a mobile fulcrum.

The harmonic scalpel is promising technology that has become popular in open (traditional) radial artery harvest. It consists of a generator/blade system in which the blade vibrates at 55 000 Hz, denaturing proteins to divide and seal side branches. This is appealing in that no clips are required to ligate the side branches. Scanning electron microscopy has demonstrated less lateral thermal damage when compared to *monopolar* electrocautery in vessels harvested by the open (*not* endoscopic) technique [8]. Harmonic shears are the most recent advance in harmonics technology. This instrument consists of an unprotected harmonic blade and an insulated blade in a scissors configuration. Theoretically, the possibility of endothelial injury with this system may exist, based upon the inherent design of the instrumentation, as the fulcrum for control remains at the wrist incision. As one works more proximally up the forearm there is loss of control which can diminish the ability to maintain a safe distance from the radial artery during side-branch division.

█ Clinical experience

From November 2001 to July 2002, we successfully harvested 54 radial arteries endoscopically in 50 patients (4 bilateral) utilizing the Vasoview Endoscopic Vessel Harvesting System coupled with the "tourniquet technique". All but one of the harvested arteries were deemed suitable for use as a bypass conduit. There was one artery successfully harvested but found to have significant atherosclerotic plaquing and thus not felt to be acceptable for grafting. Our tourniquet time averaged 36.7 minutes (range 23 to 49 minutes) and all radial artery grafts were demonstrated to be patent by Doppler analysis at completion of grafting. During 30 day follow-up, no patient required readmission for post-CABG coronary syndromes that would have required cardiac catheterization.

We experienced very few complications in the donor arm, and all were minor. No patient experienced symptoms of vascular compromise or hand ischemia. At 30 day follow-up, one

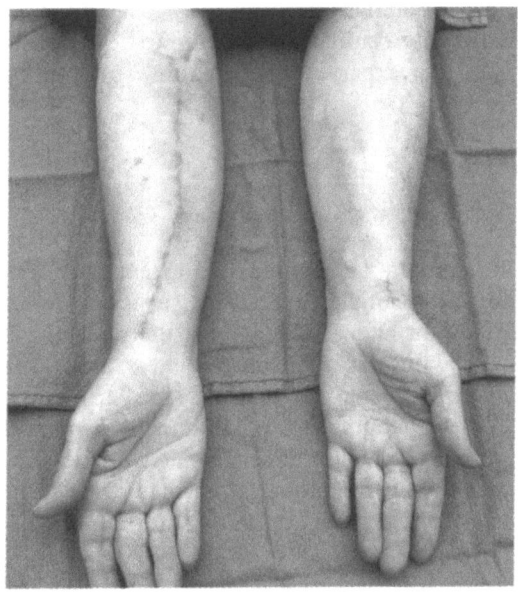

Fig. 1. Patient who underwent bilateral radial artery harvesting utilizing the open (right arm) and endoscopic (left arm) techniques 7 days after coronary bypass surgery

patient demonstrated sensory loss in the distribution of the superficial branch of the radial nerve and one patient had an exacerbation of pre-existing carpal tunnel syndrome. No patient manifested sensory loss in the lateral antebrachial cutaneous nerve distribution. As with endoscopic vein harvest, it was common to see ecchymosis in the tissues of the arm. However, there were no arm hematomas, and no adjunct procedures were required to control venous or arterial bleeding. Wound healing was uneventful, and there were no post-operative wound infections.

Our initial experience has been with bipolar electrocautery, and in our first 50 patients, we have found this to be a safe, reproducible technique. Although subjective, it is our impression that there is less vasospasm than we had encountered with the "open" harvest technique. One might argue that the sole benefit on endoscopic radial artery harvest is cosmetic (see Fig 1). However, we have found patient satisfaction to be extremely high, much as has been our experience with endoscopic vein harvest.

Summary

Recent data have stimulated a renewed interest in the radial artery as a conduit for bypass surgery. We have described a technique for endoscopic harvest that is applicable to all patients in which the surgeon contemplates radial artery use. Our initial experience suggests that the radial artery can be removed safely and yields an excellent conduit for bypass. Provided one is experienced with endoscopic techniques in vein harvest, the added learning curve is minimal. This technique offers significant benefits over the more traditional "open" harvest.

References

1. Acar G et al (1992) Revival of the radial artery for coronary artery bypass grafting. Ann Thorac Surg 54:652–660
2. Arciero RA et al (1996) The effect of tourniquet use in anterior cruciate ligament reconstruction: a prospective randomized study. Am J Sports Med 24:758–764
3. Carpentier A et al (1973) The aorta-to-coronary radial artery bypass graft: a technique avoiding pathological changes in grafts. Ann Thorac Surg 16:111–121
4. Carpentier A et al, Discussion of Geha et al (1975) Selection of coronary bypass anatomic, physiologic, and angiographic considerations of vein and mammary grafts. J Thorac Cardiovasc Surg 70:404–431
5. Curtis JJ et al (1975) Intimal hyperplasia: a cause of radial artery aorto-coronary bypass graft failure. Ann Thorac Surg 20:628–635
6. Hood JM, Lubahn JD (1994) Bipolar coagulation at different energy levels: effect on patency. Microsurgery 15(8):594–597
7. Kirkley A et al (2000) Tourniquet versus no tourniquet use in routine knee arthroscopy: a perspective, double-blind, randomized clinical trial. Arthroscopy 16:121–126
8. Lamm P, Juchem G, Weyrich P et al (2000) The harmonic scalpel: optimizing the quality of mammary artery bypass. Ann Thorac Surg 69:1833–1835
9. Tatoulis J et al (1999) The radial artery as a graft for coronary revascularization: techniques and follow-up. Advances in Cardiac Surgery 11:99–128
10. Tatoulis J et al (2002) The radial artery in coronary surgery: a 5-year experience-clinical and angiographic results. Ann Thorac Surg 73:143–148
11. Uchida A, Hachberg J, Terada Y (1998) Endoscopic harvesting of radial artery graft for coronary artery bypass. Ann Plast Surg 41(5):459–463
12. Wakai MB et al (2001) Pneumatic tourniquets in extremity surgery. J Am Acad Orthop Surg 9:345–351